*Bottom High to the Crowd*

# Bottom High
# to the Crowd

by Mary Phraner Warren
and Don Kirkendall

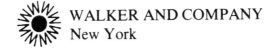 WALKER AND COMPANY
New York

First published in the United States of America in 1973 by the Walker Publishing Company, Inc.

Published simultaneously in Canada by Fitzhenry & Whiteside, Limited, Toronto.

ISBN: 0-8027-0409-3

Library of Congress Catalog Card Number: 72-95742

Printed in the United States of America.

*To my mother and wife*
*who diligently have been*
*my inspiration*

1749039

THE hospital was a big place, drab, scary, crammed with strangers and bad smells. Fresh blood, vomit, urine, soap, hospital linen, the uninviting aroma of creamed asparagus left cold and rejected on many of the trays going back to the kitchen—all these and many more were glued together by the astringent odor of antiseptic.

This was my third and, although I did not know it yet, my last visit.

Mom had brought me on the night train from our farm in eastern South Dakota. She would keep me company for two or three days while I settled into the hospital routine. Then she would return to take care of Dad and my two older brothers, Floyd and Jack.

The exciting memory of the two-hundred-mile night ride took the edge off the dismay I felt at being in the hospital once again. We'd even had meals on the train. Dining car prices were, as Mother said, always "outlandish" so we'd boarded the train bearing a picnic supper in one shoebox and a picnic breakfast of hard-boiled eggs, oranges, and bread and butter in another.

All night long I'd awakened at various times to look out the window of my bottom berth at the scenery flying by. The porter came to wake us early. He lifted me into an empty seat while he unmade our berths.

"There you go, sonny. He's pretty lightweight for a ten year old, isn't he, ma'am? We'll be in Glascow, Minnesota, in an hour. I'll carry the boy down the steps if you can manage your bags."

It began then, the feeling of being treated like a thing. In the next hour and a half, it grew steadily worse.

We took a taxi to the hospital and there an attendant plunked me into a wheelchair and pushed me in to the admitting desk. The wretched conglomeration of smells assailed my nostrils.

A familiar routine by now. While Mom answered a few questions, I was issued a nightie and a breech clout. Next I was taken, via elevator, to the isolation unit. Here I must remain until my "clear report" came back.

"Never mind," Mom comforted before she left to spend the night at her sister Maud's. "You're older now, Don. This year you'll be on the Big Boys' Ward. It may be more fun. No doubt some of the friends you made last time'll be back."

She left. I was stuck in a high bed in the little glass-enclosed room. Nobody to talk to, nothing to look at, nothing to do.

Presently the door opened. A nurse came in with a cheery smile pasted on her face. The smile disappeared as soon as I made the mistake of looking too eagerly at the basket of toys in her arms.

"You may select one thing to play with. Only one. And," she added in a severe tone, "remember, if you break it there'll be no more tomorrow."

She had not bothered to scan my chart. Since I was not a new boy but an old one returning, I was used to the stupid rule. The toys in the basket did not interest me anyway. I saw at a glance most were the same old battered things. The one puzzle I had not seen before had some pieces missing.

Haphazardly, I chose a small blue metal plane. One propeller was off but no matter. It would serve me well enough in my interior flight.

Once again, I was being forced to split into two people. The one here in the hospital bed was the puny, immobile kid from a farm in South Dakota who had no control over his own destiny.

I'd seen animals taken to be butchered. That is how I felt whenever the doctors looked me over in their impersonal, professional manner and discussed "my case." In their eyes I had no more personality than a hunk of beef or pork.

But there was, too, that unseen child who, in spite of distance and the terrific pull of the hospital, struggled to remain part of a life to which he would return one day.

When I first came to the hospital, at the age of seven, I had developed a special vehicle to carry me wherever I wished to go. The vehicle was not my wheelchair, which had become so much a part of me at home, but my imagination.

Nothing a doctor or nurse could say or do was ever able to remove its control from me.

After three days in the isolation unit, I would be moved to the ward. Here, at least, would be a bit of diversion and the companionship of other boys. But I knew from previous experience that here, too, I would face cruelty, boredom, days that would pass eternally empty while I lay in bed and wondered what was going on at home.

Incarcerated as we were, it was difficult to mark the passage of time. We lost track of the days and weeks and months. It was winter now, but somehow I would know when the chinook was blowing in South Dakota.

The feeling throbbed in my bones. When it happened, I had the satisfaction of knowing I need only close my eyes in order to become the other Don and thereby watch it work its magic.

11

Winter vanished in that wind. Not in a week but in a matter of hours. It could make tall snowbanks disappear overnight. When the chinook blew, it seemed like spring had taken a deep breath and exhaled. It seemed like spring must be telling winter, "It's my turn now, leave!"

In bed, in the room smelling of bedpans and lysol, I would think about it. The air must be sweet at home. Wedges of geese would be honking north across the sky. No doubt my brothers, Floyd and Jack, would be whooping and hollering because, finally, they could get free of the house and play in the mud.

I pictured them, boots heavy with the gummy substance, trying to scrape it off at the back door so they wouldn't mark up Mom's clean kitchen floor.

You don't know mud unless you know gumbo, that yellow-red, claylike stuff that sticks to anything that makes contact with it early in the spring when the snows begin to melt.

Buggies, wagons, farm machinery, and cars sunk several inches and got mired. Even Dad's almost indestructible flivver proved no match for gumbo.

The chinook held promises, promises of planting time, the greening of the earth, a good harvest. The farmers, their skin creased by wind and sun, stood straighter. Their hearts swelled with a renewed faith. Maybe the land would not cheat them this time. Maybe it would give them what they wanted, a living.

Surely this would be a bumper year for wheat and corn!

Dad was a tenant farmer. During the worst years of drought and dust and grasshoppers, circumstances led him to try other occupations for a time. At heart, though, he was a farmer.

Every few years we moved around the eastern part of the state. The house of my dreams was the one I loved best, the one situated on the old Hanson place between Woonsocket and Cuthbert. Cuthbert consisted of little more than a grain elevator, a store, a post office, and a church. For Saturday night sprees we drove to Woonsocket.

12

Except for a cottonwood here and there, or an occasional windbreak of poplar, the land boasted no trees. Our brown house stuck out on the horizon like a slab of molasses taffy. Its color was unusual for that part of the country. For miles around, every other house was painted white.

The house had character. People who stuck through dust storms, drought, and grasshopper plagues had character too. And, as for Dad, he *was* a character. He and the dogs were the characters I loved best.

There were others—my Grandfather Merrit, the tall, bald auctioneer known around the county as a natty dresser. And my mother and old Otto Proudhammer and Darcy Collens. But Dad and the dogs came first, to my mind.

Dad had a short and stocky build. His grim countenance made him look like the meanest man in eastern South Dakota. Underneath the surly crust, one could find a surprisingly gentle creature.

His favorite phrase,"son of a bitch," took on a variety of meanings. It depended entirely upon the situation at hand, and the tone of Dad's voice.

At times Dad said son of a bitch as tenderly as a bridegroom says "I love you." He crooned it like a lullaby, as well as spitting it out when his temper grew short and things weren't going his way. He never used the phrase on another man. It was reserved for animals and inanimate objects.

He came out with those four words in the manner other people muttered gee or golly. He tackled his machinery with them, and his dogs. The dogs understood. All of them adored my father.

Our farm dogs bore no resemblance to the leisure class city canines I'd seen from the taxicab on the way to the hospital. They were a far cry from the haughty, purebred show dogs in magazine pictures, and different, too, from the happy-go-lucky Heinz variety people kept as family pets in town.

A farm dog might be a child's companion, yes. In his spare time. First he had work to do. Besides that, a Kirkendall dog knew his place. He never set foot inside the house. Not if Mom saw him.

Our dog was familiar with his assigned tasks. To begin with, he was a watch dog. Nobody taught him this skill. It was a basic part of his being. We lived in a very rural area. Frontier days were not far in the past. Much of the ruggedness of pioneer life persisted. Farming was mostly on a small-sized, family scale. Gangs of outlaws roamed the land.

One of these outlaw bands could easily tear down a dirt road with the sheriff hot on their heels, swerve suddenly into a corn-field, and get lost.

Unless he happened to be on the spot at the right moment, a dog couldn't do a blessed thing about that. But let him scent a stranger, a panhandler for instance, approaching the farmyard and he'd let his family know in a hurry.

Our dog knew how to keep the chickens in line. With a yapping dog around, not one poor little banty dared adventure from the yard. With gusto, he saw to it no hawk or coyote sneaked in to capture a meal.

At milking time who rounded up the cows and brought them home to the shed? The dog of course. When there were sheep to be herded, that was his duty too.

The smartest dog we ever owned was Nick, a medium-sized brown dog with white scruff and long tail curling tight up over his back. A nondescript dog was Nick, but he loved us three boys something terrible.

A lump came into my throat whenever I got to thinking about Nick. I could close my eyes and find him prancing along my eyelids, real as real.

Rain or shine, in summer heat or in the bitterness of winter, Nick slept on top of a haystack near the barn. When he got too cold he'd burrow completely into the hay. A passerby could see nothing but a black nose sticking out for air.

Nick kept a vigilant eye on Mom's chickens, but when it came to bringing in the cows at night he was apt to get overly

14

ambitious. At times he hamstrung them with a vicious nip in the ankle. Those were the times Dad muttered son of a bitch in an *un*conventional tone and cured him with a rock.

The dog knew what the deal was and took it easy for a while.

One family living north of the Hanson place owned a dog that was half coyote. This half-breed was an outsider to all other dogs. They were unable to tolerate the coyote smell. One day he ventured onto our property. Nick took him in a bloody battle and he never returned.

We liked to tease Nick by filling an old inner tube with water. This we attached to our artesian well. Frustrated, he'd tug and battle this enemy until . . . *pow* . . . one of his sharp teeth would penetrate the rubber, sending a fountain of water into the air. He'd back off yelping, but he liked games as much as any of us kids. He never did get tired of this one. If he got a good drenching one day, he'd be ready to have a go at the tire the very next time Floyd filled one up.

His real intelligence came out when we hunted for gophers. These small brown creatures were such pests in the cornfields that there was a bounty on their tails.

By the tender age of six, any farm boy was a crackerjack shot with a rifle. Every child wanted to collect the three cents a tail offered for gophers.

This was the way we did it. First Jack and Floyd took the precaution of tying me in the buggy. Polio had left me with useless legs and only one good arm. I could get a bead on a gopher though, with my twenty-two. By propping the gun against my weak arm and using the good one, I'd learned to shoot as well as my brothers.

When I'd been properly strapped in, the boys lugged over a barrel full of water. This was fastened to the back of the buggy. The barrel had a spigot on it.

Off we'd go, across the fields, stopping only to open and close barbed wire fences when we came to them.

Laughing and shouting, we'd flood those gophers out of their holes. They were plentiful and easy to catch. Often we clubbed them to death instead of wasting good shells on them. Then we hacked off the tails so we could turn them in and collect the bounty. After we made a catch we rode off, leaving half a dozen poor little corpses strewn on the ground behind the buggy.

A gopher is a hardy creature. It soon became apparent we did not actually kill every gopher we clubbed. The ones we stunned lived to run again and this is where Nick's brains showed up. When he accompanied us on our forays, he knew enough not to bring us a tailless gopher!

Nick had one favorite game he played where he finally was the loser. In the dead of winter in our part of South Dakota, snow piled pretty high. Cars and wagons carved deep ruts. As winter wore on toward spring, the ruts got deeper and deeper and the snowbanks on either side grew higher until they were well over a man's head

Nick had a passion for chasing cars, especially the mailman's car. Seems like he considered an automobile to be a threatening kind of animal. Each day he lay down in the snowy ruts, ears flattened out, tensed to spring. As soon as the car went by, he made a flying leap and barked it all the way to our mailbox.

His timing was excellent. He relied on his own agility to get out of the way. But one day his paws slipped in the icy rut. He was killed.

Dad and another farmer were on hand and watched it happen. The mailman felt so dreadful he almost cried. He got out of his car and said, "Kirk, I killed your dog."

"Son of a bitch," muttered Dad who felt as dismayed as the others to see Nick's still body lying bloody in the snow. "Son of a bitch, it was his own durn fault. Don't think anymore about it."

From childhood on, my father had had this stark realism bred into him. It came out in the way he dealt with a dead dog, a creature he'd been particularly fond of, too.

It came out, also, in the way he handled a small son in a wheelchair. Whenever I was around Dad, I could be certain of one thing. He was not a sentimental man but underneath that gruff, muleskinner talk of his, there was a kind heart. He couldn't scare me with his grim looks and wild phrases.

If he pitied me, he never showed it. That, of course, was why I loved him.

Dad treated me like a regular boy. He called me Don instead of Donnie, thereby adding to my stature. Whenever I needed it, he gave me a hiding.

One day Jack dared me to take a crack at the new oil drum with my twenty-two.

"If you hit between the first and second ring," my brother volunteered grandly, "I'll take the beating for you."

I hit it between the first and second ring all right. But where was Jack? Out behind the manure pile, laughing fit to kill. Dad gave it to me proper and it was a long time before I forgave Jack for such a lowdown brotherly trick.

My father had little formal education. He was born of sweat-and-muscle parents, pioneer stock who did not hold with such truck.

"Education's all right, but you got to make a living with your hands." That's what they told him. He'd been through five grades, but he'd read more books than many a man who went on to college.

He was quiet, Dad was. But when he said something, brother, he meant it! It took a long time to get him riled up. After you finally succeeded, look out! You could count on him remaining that way until he worked things through in his own mind.

His vocabulary included many words but not dishonesty. He had no comprehension of that trait.

Dad refused to put the family in debt to own a piece of land. That was why he was a tenant farmer.

Trusting? Often he left his keys in the car and went off about his business for a few hours. He did it in the small towns and also in the bigger ones like Mitchell or Sioux City.

"Never can tell when a fellow may come along and need to move it," was his reasoning.

Since he did not bother to lock our house, we might come home from an all-day jaunt and discover a note propped against the sugar bowl on the kitchen table:

"Hi Kirk. Stopped by and had lunch. Where were you?" signed Bill.

There developed a special camaraderie between Dad and me. His abrupt manner contained more healing in it than the prayers of the preacher who stopped by now and then to lay his hand heavily on my shoulder and utter sonorous platitudes like "Poor poor little Donnie."

If poor poor little Donnie could have managed it, he would have kicked that preacher man in the shins.

I hated to be called Donnie. Besides that, I didn't feel so very poor whenever Dad was hauling me around in the seat of the hayrack, regaling me with bawdy tales of gangster bands in Canada.

As a young man, Dad had homesteaded there. Whether or not his stories were true or half-true, or utterly false, I never discovered. Certainly they made good listening.

Nor did I wallow in self-pity when Dad shoved my wheelchair down the main street of Woonsocket on a Sunday morning, farting to beat the band. Nobody could fart like my father. I'll lay a bet to it any day.

He could do it any time he wanted to so he did it all the time. Not to be obnoxious, of course. He had a mind of his own and he thought it was funny.

Of course he embarrassed Mom to tears, making such an inappropriate noise en route to church. She did not have the courage to turn and see which of her astonished Christian bretheren might be taking in the scene. At first she'd stiffen up her back and order him primly, in a low voice:

"Kirk, stop that! Kirk, shut up!"

18

At that Dad would go to bigger and better extremes. Pressing her lips together in a thin line of annoyance, Mom continued to reprimand him. At last, in sheer exasperation, she'd flare up with a touch of wry humor:

"You could probably play 'Yankee Doodle' with that."

Just short of the church, he'd stop. He had discovered, long ago, the easiest way of handling a woman.

When Mom hollered or fussed, he knew enough not to holler back. But he refused to do whatever she asked if he did not feel like it. He never walked away. He'd answer her questions, sure enough, but add no extra comment.

When my father grew quiet, you could feel his silence like a stone.

Iowa born, Mom had a mind of her own, too. In the evening, when chores were done, she lit the kerosene lamp and read us Bible stories and many of the classics. Immersed in *Tom Sawyer* or one of Kipling's *Jungle Books*, we traveled worlds away from our snowbound house on the plains of South Dakota.

By day Mom did her share of heavy farm work. She helped with the haying in summertime. At times she drove the cultivator. She took care of the chickens and hogs. She baked bread, churned, washed our heavy work-a-day clothing in her hand-crank washing machine, and hung it out on the line to dry.

We had no electricity in our house, and no "ice box." We kept our dairy products in caves. The caves were simply holes in the ground, deep ones like root cellars but a little nicer, where we could keep things cool.

Sometimes in the hottest weather we set food in a pail and dropped it to the water level in the cistern to keep it from spoiling.

One thing my mother refused to do . . . gardening. She took no pride in messing around with tomatoes and cucumbers and squash. To her way of thinking, it was a man's job. So my oldest brother, Floyd, and Dad ended up in the garden and, whenever possible, Jack helped.

Sometimes my straight-laced, Bible reading mother turned out to be full of surprises to those of us who thought we knew her well.

Once our neighbor's geese meddled with our garden too often to suit Mom. She issued a terse warning to their owner:

"Keep your critters off our property. Next time I see'm I'll shoot."

The geese challenged her statement the next day. Mom reached for the rifle, took aim, and fired. She was as good a shot as the rest of us so the case was closed.

It was Mom who encouraged me on each of these horrendous trips to the hospital in Minnesota. She had faith the big city doctors could help me walk again.

After months of separation, I could lie in bed and, with eyes closed, conjure up a picture of Mother in her faded cotton wash dress and apron. A picture so true to life it was difficult to comprehend she was not at my side but actually two hundred miles away.

I was two Dons, but mostly the hidden one who bore within him this ripening golden world of memory. In it I could laugh and sing and do my share of family chores, shoot Fourth of July firecrackers, carve Jack o'Lanterns, steal watermelons with the rest of the gang, get sick on the vile cigarettes we rolled for ourselves behind the outhouse, shoot gophers, ride the hayrack with Dad, or play the games Jack and I had invented to pass the long winter days while we waited for spring to come.

"Tsk! And how're we doing today?" A young, red-headed nurse coming on afternoon duty paused briefly to poke a thermometer between my lips. She did not wait for an answer but bustled on to the next boy in the bed beside mine. And the next and the next.

I watched her go. She was one of the prettier ones, sparkly and full of life. In the spring she'd be getting married and then she could go home to smalltown life and be a housewife and have children of her own. I knew because I'd overheard her showing her engagement ring to a bunch of less fortunate nurses amid Oh's and Ah's.

Never mind. I had learned to go away, too. And I needed no train to take me. Whenever Miss Blood (that was the name of the crankiest one of all) or any of the cool, efficient nurses came in to chide us for getting noisy, I could, in one split second, depart into my other world and be free.

## two

THREE memories I had of the years before I became sick with polio. Memories of running and climbing. The rest was as blurred as the sky before a blizzard.

Once I ran away from home. I was only three years old. Floyd and Jack, big boys of seven and five, rode horseback to the country school two miles down the road from the farm.

Each morning I watched them go, both astride the same horse. And each morning I was overcome by that left-out feeling common to the youngest child.

How I longed to swing my own lunchpail full of bread and butter, apples, and leftover pheasant! How I yearned to be the proud possessor of important items like a Reader, a dogeared Speller, a fistful of pencils, a tablet of clean, ruled paper.

And so I took it into my head to investigate that mysterious place called *school*.

As soon as the horse was out of sight one day, I set off as fast as my legs could carry me. Behind me I could hear the thump-

thump, thump-thump of Mom's churn. Dad was out working some place on the farm.

Determined to reach the schoolhouse, I did not pause once to blow a dandelion or pick up a rock. I held no conversation, this morning, with gopher or pheasant. I covered at least half of the distance between house and school before Dad caught up with me.

He'd been getting sand in a borrowed truck. Seeing me trot by at a fast clip, he figured I must be up to mischief.

He stopped and flung open the car door and hoisted me into the high seat. His lips twitched in a ghost of a smile.

"Where in tarnation did you think you were headed, Don?"

"School," I whispered in a small voice, hoping to avoid a walloping if I leveled with him. "I wanted to go to school like Floyd and Jack."

"Plenty of time for that later," was all he said. "Right now you better come home and have a cup of milk and go play."

I remembered another time. A blissful late spring evening. My brothers must have considered me old enough to tag along with the gang. Of course they were pushed to do so since Mom expected them to keep an eye on me while she busied herself with scrubbing the kitchen floor.

Supper had been over a long time ago. Dusk fell as we became engrossed in a rousing game of Hide and Seek. The older children had longer legs than I. They bounded over the field like jack rabbits. Even the twin girls from the neighboring farm were ahead of me. I did my best to keep up with them so they'd allow me to stay in the game. On top of the potato cellar, I took a header. I caught my knee on a nail tearing out a nickel-sized chunk of flesh.

The game came to an abrupt halt with my screeching.

"Shut up!" commanded Floyd. Impatiently, he tried to mop the blood up with his handkerchief. "Aw come on and let Mom fix it. I guess she'll have to douse it with turpentine or something."

The third memory was one of running a race. Those vast and treeless stretches of South Dakota farmland gave any child an uncontrollable urge to whoop it up. No jungle gyms or civilized play equipment for us! From dawn until dark, we got our exercise by tearing all over creation in a buggy or on foot.

Running races was a favorite pastime. One day I figured out how I could make myself go faster. All I needed to do was to put one foot as far in front of the other as possible.

First one foot, then the other. One foot, reach. The other foot . . . reeeeach!

But there came an afternoon when, quite without warning, the carefree world of running was lost to me forever except in dreams.

The thing I enjoyed best on a blistering summer afternoon was to climb up the side of the cattle feeder. Up over the splintery slats my four-year-old legs would clamber. Up and up. From that height, I could view the gently rolling land for miles. Various farms were laid out in a panorama before me like a child's toy . . . miniature houses and barns, silos, windmills and fields, grazing cattle, the schoolhouse, railroad tracks and weathered gray depot, grain elevator, general store, the church with its thin spire gleaming in the blazing sun.

What an exhilarating feeling to be able to see it like that, all in one swoop! I was king of the world.

One normally thinks of blue as a cool color. But this day was so hot that the end-of-the-summer Dakota sky burned with a metallic brilliance. The blue color dazzled so it made my eyes water. When a flock of crows flew overhead, I had to squinch my eyes shut to see them.

"Caw!" I called in a loud voice. "Caw, caw! You better fly off or Mom'll be out to getcha with her shotgun."

Actually it was the newly planted corn, soft and sweet and still in the milk, that crows demolished each year. In summer when it had become hard and dry, they feasted mainly on thousands of bugs—beetles, cutworms, grasshoppers . . . This beneficial work of theirs failed to endear them to the farmers since they'd first proved themselves to be pesky, obnoxious birds by destroying the young corn.

During our leanest years, we never got hungry enough to try baking four and twenty of the huge black birds with glossy blue-black wings in a pie. That was because pheasant was always in abundance. But we certainly did use the crows for target practice.

No doubt about it, they were clever birds. When they were getting ready to raid our newly planted cornfields, often they would think to post a sentinel to warn them of approaching danger.

At times one of the big fellows taunted Mom by perching saucily on a fencepost so close she couldn't possibly miss him with the first crack of her gun. But he had made certain to have a cow between himself and the weapon. He seemed to know Mom wouldn't fire for fear of hitting one of her own cows.

"Dratted bird!" she fumed. "Robbing the cornfield isn't the worst those crows do. They're . . . they're *carniverous*! They steal my chickens."

She was protective of her chickens. The egg money and the chicken money belonged to her to squander on a bit of cloth or a new book to read to the family at night.

After a while I got tired of hollering at the crows so I set to flicking the little green worms out of the straw in the feeder. Sweet clover hay in a hot Dakota sun . . . I hung there inhaling it and thinking I'd never known anything so delicious.

From the other side of the cattle feeder, I could hear our hired man, John, pitching hay into the trough below so the cattle could eat it.

John was more than hired help. He was good company, and fun to be around, exceedingly patient with the three of us boys. If we bothered him, he never let on. He was little more than a big boy himself, and we considered him part of our family while we lived on that farm. Naturally he felt this gave him the right to reprimand us or spank us or boss us whenever necessary.

Today he cautioned me, "Watch it, Donald. You're a small tyke to be up so high."

"I'm OK," I yelled back. "John, how do the little green

worms get into the hay? Do they climb all the way from the ground?''

"How would I know such a thing?'' he laughed good-naturedly. "Donald! Didn't I just finish telling you to watch out? There now, I ain't gonna tell you again. *Hang on!*''

It was too late. I'd already fallen.

I hit the sun-baked ground with a thud and lay there, momentarily stunned. John hurried over and picked me up, feeling me carefully with his strong fingers before he heaved a sigh of relief.

"No broken bones, you lucky kid! Didn't even draw a drop of blood.''

But he continued to peer at me worriedly since I looked as white as milk, and shaken.

"Must've knocked your breath clean out. Come on, then. We better go in and tell your Maw.''

He hoisted me into his brawny arms and carted me off to the house.

"Tsk.'' Mom clicked her tongue against her teeth. "What were you doing on that high old thing in this heat? Lie down on my big bed for a while, Don. A little nap'll do you good.''

She went back to the pile of mending at her treadle sewing machine. Drowsily I listened to the whirr until at last I drifted off to sleep.

My nap turned into a nightmare without beginning or end. The bugs I'd been playing with on the cattle feeder grew to monstrous size.

"They're after me, they're after me!'' I moaned in my sleep. "Those bugs keep on biting me. Oh Mom, make them stop!''

Her cool, rough hand smoothed away the perspiration on my forehead. "Hush, Donald. It isn't the fall that's doing this to you. You've come down with a bad fever. Flu, I think. They have it over to the Olson farm, so that must be what it is. Hush, Don, there are no bugs.''

"Yes there are, Mom. Really! They're after me! Oh Mom, my throat hurts just awful.''

Hours passed. I moved in and out of that terrible nightmare. A strong wind had risen at sunset, followed by heavy rain. Mom and Dad tiptoed in and out of the bedroom, feeling my burning forehead and conferring with one another in anxious whispers.

Soberly, Floyd and Jack scrubbed their faces at the wash basin and did their teeth and went to bed with a minimum of noise. Mom hardly had to hush them. It was obvious I was terribly sick.

Once I heard her cranking the phone to get through to the family doctor in town. I saw her bulky form in the doorway of the bedroom as she said in a low voice:

"Kirk, I told him how sick the boy is. You know what he told me? 'Give the kid a couple of aspirins to break the fever. He'll come round. I can't possibly get out on a night like this.''

By this time my throat hurt so bad I couldn't swallow, and my arms and legs ached so I could hardly lift them. When Mom held a cup to my dry lips, my teeth clinked hard against the rim and water dribbled down the front of my pajamas.

By morning I was in a semicoma.

When next I opened my eyes, a nurse in a starched uniform hovered near my bed with a spoon. It wasn't my folks' big bed but a high metal one with siderails on it. The sheets had a peculiar antiseptic smell that I did not like.

I was in the hospital in Mitchell, twenty-five miles from home.

"Now be a good child and take this medicine, Donald, " coaxed the nurse. "If you swallow it, I'll bring you ice cream. Or jello. Whatever you like."

"I'll take jelly," I whispered weakly. My voice wouldn't come out right. It sounded faint and separate from me, floating on the air as if it belonged to another boy.

The aches had disappeared. I felt no pain now but only an enormous, indescribable weakness. It overcame me. I could not raise my hand off the blanket to reach for the spoon and saucer of jello the nurse soon brought. Nor could I sit up or even turn my head. But I was too sick to be frightened.

I did not yet know that every muscle in my body, except for my eyeballs, was paralyzed.

"You've had polio," explained the nurse while she fed the jello to me. "Your mother is right here. She dozed off for a few minutes, poor thing. She's been staying in the hospital but you were so sick she couldn't catch a wink of sleep until now. My, for a small boy you had us worried!"

"Let me feed him," said a mellow voice. "You go take care of your other patients."

Mom bent over and brushed my cheek with a kiss.

"You're better today, Donald. The nurse is right. You've had us pretty worried, but you're doing OK."

The voice was hers but she looked like a stranger without her apron on. Besides, her face had a greyish cast and the merriness was gone out of her eyes. A combination of fear and worry and lack of sleep had turned them into two gaping holes.

Was this Mom? I felt confused.

Lest I sense her pain, she straightened her shoulders. She sounded firm when she said gently, "You'll be getting well quicker if you eat. I'll have nurse bring you some beef broth and a straw."

All at once I caught a whiff of her special mothery kind of a smell—impossible to capture in words because so much went into it—hair, skin, dress, sweat, soap mixed together in a way that was *her*. With a sigh of recognition, I closed my eyes and went back to sleep.

Days and nights faded into one another. Mostly I slept. My waking moments seemed vague, the only real thing being the constant parade of doctors and nurses and internes who tiptoed in and out of the room, consulting charts, whispering to each other about my condition.

"He's holding his own. Nothing to do but wait," they told my mother. "Perhaps some day we'll discover a cure for infantile paralysis. Right now there's nothing."

"Nothing but prayer," murmured my mother in a voice so

28

low they scarcely heard. A stubborn woman, she was not about to give up.

The year was 1927. The world had radios and airplanes, automobiles, pasteurized milk, anesthetics to relieve pain. It had vaccines for small pox and diptheria, but none for polio.

My folks had never before come up against a disease untreatable with the simplest of home remedies.

Boiled skunk's oil was a favorite panacea for rheumatic aches and pains. And turpentine supposedly had great power to heal. Dad used a smelly mixture of turpentine and lard on his castrated hogs. If a horse happened to come down with boils or a child stumbled into a hornets' nest, he packed them with mud. Eucalyptus oil was another favorite, especially for colds in the chest. Dad once cured a hog dying of pneumonia by shutting it up in a room and steaming it with a concoction of eucalyptus oil and boiling water. His rule seemed infallible: the smellier, the more vile-tasting the medicine, the better the cure.

That may have been the main reason we boys did our best to stay well.

My mother's frequent reports by telephone from the hospital in Mitchell made him feel terribly helpless. The power had gone out of his cures. He, too, could do nothing but wait.

At first nobody expected me to pull through. Nobody except Mom. She continued to bombard the gates of heaven with prayers. She had too much respect for the Almighty to order Him around, but she did a fair amount of pleading.

I remained a motionless scrap of skin and bones. It was anyone's guess whether or not I would ever sit up or walk again, but I was alive. In a few weeks, Dad appeared at the hospital to take me back to the farm.

The harvest had been good. As he lifted me into his arms, he remarked casually, "I've a surprise for you outside, Donald." He tried to smile, in spite of his worry over me. "Wait till you see!"

He'd bought a shiny new four-door Chevrolet, a blue

one. I was awed. But a crestfallen look passed over Mom's face.

"Kirk, we'll be having so many bills! You shouldn't have done it!"

"Had to. How else will we be able to take Don places when we go? I don't aim to stay home while he's getting better and it looks as if it may take him some time. I sold some of our live-stock, Missus. Got pretty good money for 'em, too."

Mom slid her fingers over the sleek back of the car seat and her face brightened. "Anyway, it *is* beautiful."

There were very few shiny, new, *beautiful* things on our farm.

Life went on. Nothing had changed, yet, in truth, everything had changed. The clock ticked out the hours in its same old place on the kitchen shelf, my brothers banged in and out of the house, helping Dad with the chores. Mom scalded the basins and milk cans, strained the milk, and carried it out to the caves until Dad got around to carting much of it into town to sell. She moved in and out of the house, feeding her chickens, baking, churning, sewing. Her own chores were time-consuming, and now she had an invalid to care for in addition to everything else. But it was not her way to hurry through the day. She merely did what had to be done.

I could not turn my own small body in bed. Someone had to do it for me. Mom folded a clean sheet in fourths and set me on it. When I needed to be turned, she gathered the four corners of the sheet with me inside it, hammock fashion, and rolled me over. When I soiled the bed she washed my sheets in her hand-crank washing machine and hung them out to dry.

Somebody had to sit by my bed three times a day and feed me. I must be lifted on and off the bedpan, bathed, dressed, con-stantly attended. If a fly landed on my nose, I had no way of moving to brush it off. I could not hold up my head. Whenever I was propped or held in an upright position, it fell forward on my chest.

30

Floyd and Jack took turns feeding and entertaining me. But they were boisterous, active youngsters, eager to be out of the house much of the time. Dad was as busy as any other farmer, and Floyd preferred helping with the "mens work" to being my nursemaid.

It was Jack, a sturdy fiesty little boy with horned-rimmed specs who eventually took on the task of watching over me and playing with me. Jack and Mother.

Mother boasted to the rest of the family at the supper table whenever there was the slightest progress.

"Kirk, Floyd, Jack—did you notice how Don can move the fingers on his left hand? That's good, isn't it!"

The paralysis was slow to leave.

Bills came in. Retrieving them from the R.F.D. box, Mom glanced at them with a grimace and a sigh. Then she propped them on a kitchen shelf near the salt cellars where Dad might not notice them until he'd had a good hot dinner.

With Mom, tears came as easily to the surface as smiles. Now and then when she thought I was sound asleep, I watched her rocking in the chair near my bed, weeping to herself. Finally she'd fumble for the handkerchief in her apron pocket, and wipe her eyes and go out to feed the chickens.

At night in the darkened bedroom, Mom and Dad lay awake and talked.

"We'll manage somehow, Kirk."

"But how? That's what I want to know. All those bills . . ."

"You said yourself, it's a bumper crop. We may have another one next year, too."

The springs of the bed creaked as Mom's heavy body twisted and turned. "The important thing is for Donald to get better. I heard about a new young doctor in Sioux Falls. He might be able to give us some idea of what could be done . . ."

A low whistle pierced the silence. Weary from a hot day in the fields, Dad was responding with a snore.

Crisp autumn days turned to winter. Chores were done early. Mom had already lit the kerosene lamps before Dad got back from the barn. At night the wind hissed around the house and the window panes rattled. In the morning the ground outside my window smoked with frost.

Before long, Floyd and Jack would have to leave the horse at home and plod through snow to school. Mom hurried to finish the mittens and hats she was knitting from scraps of colored yarn. She pored over the Sears Roebuck catalog, trying to decide whether she could squander money for a warm jacket for Floyd.

At ten, he was shooting up. His elbows had split through the sleeves of his old blue jacket and he kept popping buttons because it had become too tight across the chest.

"I can patch your old one for Jack," she decided as she wrote the order. "It's perfectly good."

"Hey, don't I get a new one?" began Jack. But then he glanced at me and over at Mom again. "Aw, that's OK. I don't care."

Home was a warm and comforting place. I could not move around but I could hear and see and smell.

Whenever I woke up early, I lay in bed and listened to Dad getting ready to go out to take care of the stock with Floyd.

"Son of a bitch, where'd I put my *hat?*"

Dad never went anyplace without his ancient brown felt hat shoved down on his head. That hat was part of him, just as an apron was part of my mother. Once in an emergency, he rushed stark naked out of the bedroom but paused long enough to clap his hat on his head before he attended to the matter at hand.

I heard the back door click shut. Snow scrunched underfoot as Dad and Floyd headed for the barn. A little later there would be the thud-bump of milk cans and, pretty soon, the hollow bangity-clank of the metal wash basin. Mom must be filling it with roaring hot water from the "reservoir" at the back of the stove so Dad could shave.

When I heard Floyd and Jack arguing over the last drops of

maple syrup in the pitcher, I knew it must be a pancake and sausage morning.

Mom's breakfasts ran big. As often as not, *both* pancakes and fried potatoes were served, along with canned fruit of some kind, and two or three eggs apiece.

On a morning when she substituted oatmeal for pancakes, it was doused with heavy cream and a veritable blizzard of sugar. Her oatmeal had to be cooked for a long time until it became thick enough to chew. It was nothing like the thin, lumpy stuff served at the hospital.

Gradually I got well enough to be lifted from bed to couch. Now I was able to see everything that happened. I could not hold a picture book yet, but Mom found time to rest during the day, and she would sit by me and talk or read out loud.

Sometimes the neighbor ladies came for coffee. Now they had something more interesting to talk about than recipes and dress patterns. They were consumed with curiosity about my condition. They clucked over me until I grew to despise words or looks of sympathy.

The pious "Christian" kind of sympathy was the worst kind.

I was used to Mom's prayers. But when the preacher stood by the bed and prayed, his godly voice sounded very different from his everyday voice. It took on a hushed and mournful quality and made my flesh crawl.

I wanted to shout in rage, "Go away!" I didn't do it though. Mom might reach over and give me a good cuff on the ear. She didn't hold with rudeness.

Often I met the inevitable frustrations with anger or tears. But I began to discover a better way. Quite without meaning to, Dad taught me there's nothing like a good belly laugh to help a person see things in perspective. His own wit was dry, subtle. He was able to size people up in a matter of minutes.

He did not take a shine to Preacher Hagglethorpe. And the ways he handled the parson's visits were ludicrous.

One day he came back from the field to have a cigarette. His countenance turned grim when he glanced out the window.

"Son of a bitch, Don. Here comes that preacher guy with his Goddamn prayers. You better pretend to be asleep. I'll just sneak out the back door.

"By the way, if he wakes you up, tell him I've gone to Woonsocket."

## three

# 1749039

THE hard, lean dry years were upon us, the scalding summers when we lived inside an oven. No rain fell. On the southern plains, the wheat crops failed. In our corner of South Dakota, green spears of corn grew brittle and brown, too shriveled to use for anything but fodder.

Before the black blizzard of dust came a plague of grasshoppers. Monstrous in size, they swarmed in to cover the countryside. Clouds of grasshoppers descended. In front of our disbelieving eyes, they stripped an entire field of corn in a day.

On some days they were so thick in the sky they blacked out the sun. They fell into our water pails. They ate right through the clothes on the line in back of the house. When she saw that, my mother's eyes brimmed with tears. She said little as she gathered any pieces of clothing she could find without holes and attempted to scrub out the ugly brown blotches of "tobacco juice" spit by those hateful creatures.

The government provided poison with arsenic in it. Farmers

35

were instructed to catch a bunch of grasshoppers, poison them, and spread the dead bodies out on the ground. Live grasshoppers turned into cannibals. They feasted on the carcasses of others and died themselves. But then more came, and still more.

Dad had arsenic poisoning for a while, but he did not give up hope.

And then after the grasshoppers, a worse thing happened. Dust storms rolled in upon the already dry and ruined land.

Once a green, luxuriant ocean of grass had covered the Great Plains. The fibrous roots of grass had held the soil. So tenacious were those roots, the strongest winds in the driest years could not budge the earth.

The soil's humus possessed a spongelike quality. It stored enough water to feed the grass in years without rain. Long before I was born, Indians lived on the plains. They were wanderers and the plains animals, too, were wanderers. Bison, jack rabbits, coyote, antelope, gophers. Because the creatures inhabiting the land were on the move, the grass had opportunity to restore itself.

Then pioneers began to settle the plains. The pattern was broken. The building of railroads made a big difference. The ranch boom was on. And, at last, the coming of the homesteader caused the biggest change of all.

Homesteaders needed a way to protect their crops from the ranchers' cattle. Until now, cattle and sheep had roamed freely over the country. And now how could fences be built without wood or stones or hedges?

Someone thought of a way. Barbed wire fences were invented and the pattern of life on the great expanse of treeless land was changed forever. Soon every square mile of eastern South Dakota farmland was marked off with barbed wire fences. A new problem arose. The fences did keep livestock from destroying the crops. But when cattle and sheep remained in one spot, they overgrazed the land.

Years passed. And the grass no longer held the soil.

Homesteaders brought something else besides shiny rolls of

barbed wire fence. Plows. The sharp edges of their plows cut through the tough sod cover. Machines bit into the grass and plowed it under.

In time, bigger and better steel monsters . . . huge tractors . . . finished the job. The damage had been done. Farmers were plowing their fields in straight lines, laying their land open to further erosion.

But they had seen prosperous years come and go. Surely this drought would end. One day the fields would be green again. I had heard my father say this many times.

A few spits of rain would make his bleary eyes light up. For nearly two years I had been bedridden most of the time. I could see little of the havoc brought about by drought. From the couch, I watched Dad stand in the doorway, gazing at the land before him. Time and again, he yanked his small cloth sack of Bull Durham out of his trouser pocket, rolled a cigarette, and took a few puffs before shaking his fist at the sky.

"Son of a bitch, let down, will ya? Gol darn it, anyway!"

At first Mom scolded when Floyd and Jack tromped into the house without wiping their dusty feet. But, as the drought wore on, she grew quiet. There was so much dust they couldn't help bringing in some of it.

Tumbleweeds skittered down the road in the wind and occasionally I caught sight of the small eddies of dust we nicknamed "go-devils."

When Dad carried me outside for a breath of air, I coughed. The brown, dry world smelled dusty and stale. The land had a thirsty look about it, stretching parched and helpless under a cloudless sky.

The mailman stopped to shove the new Sears catalog and a fistful of bills into our box. Without a word, Dad strode over to get the bills. He took me back into the house and set me down on the couch before he handed the mail to Mom with smoldering eyes.

"Kirk!" she pleaded. "We'll find a way."

But she set the new catalog away in a drawer. I knew she would not be licking her thumb to pore over it and order fall jeans and shirts. We'd have to make do with what we had this year.

I tried to cheer Dad up with some news. For me, it was big news, bigger than droughts and crops and bills.

"I kin use my left hand now, Dad . . . look!"

"Well now, Don, that's a good sign, I'll say!" His sunburned face cracked in a tired smile. He bent to watch me make marks with a crayon on some paper.

"I kin hold a spoon of pudding without dropping it. And see how I draw good now?"

"Has the Missus been teaching you that?"

"No, I'm teaching myself. I got to do it. My other hand isn't any good."

It was my first lesson, a lesson of acceptance. Inherently, I had realized it would be a waste of energy to fight something I could not change.

But acceptance did not spell defeat. I would seek out small victories, like using my left hand.

One day after staring long at the shriveled cornfields, Dad turned to Mom.

"No telling how long she'll last. A body can never outguess a drought. But I can tell you one thing, Missus. I won't take it sitting down. This isn't any kind of life for a boy like Don. He won't get anywhere if he's buried on a dried-up farm like this his whole life long. He needs to live in town and get some schooling."

He tossed his cigarette stub to the ground, grinding it absentmindedly with the heel of his heavy work shoe.

"That's right, Kirk." Mom nodded in agreement. "But how are we going to manage it? We can't just up and leave the crops."

"Jeee—rusalem! *What* crops?" Dad glared at the corn withered beyond recognition under the merciless sun. "Why we'll probably have to end up *buying* fodder this year. When that happens, it's bad.''

He shoved his ancient hat down on his head. "I'm going in to town. Get Floyd to do the milking if I'm not back in time.''

Dark fell and there was no sign of Dad. Mom fed us our peanut butter sandwiches and got me ready for bed. It was September but the house felt as stifling as if it was back in the middle of July. It was too hot for Floyd and Jack to run around outside. Instead, they sat at the kitchen table and squabbled over a game of checkers.

"If you boys can't stop that this instant, you can both hop yourselves right into bed,'' said Mom fiercely. Then her voice turned gentle. "Here Donald.''

She set a basin of water by my bed and rinsed my perspiring face and body. She propped me carefully against a pillow in a sitting position. As usual, she planted one of her hands firmly on my chest to keep my head from falling forward.

"Let me help you brush your teeth, son. And don't you go spitting on me,'' she teased.

When I was through, she helped me lay down and set about straightening the sheets, chatting amiably as she did so.

My bath had cooled me down for a minute or two but as soon as I was in my clean pajamas and in bed, I felt hot again.

"Floyd, Jack, get over here. Time for a story.''

"Black Beauty,'' shouted Floyd. "We haven't had an animal story for ages.''

"No, Huck Finn,'' shouted Jack. He was so sweaty his glasses kept slipping down his nose. Jack had been blind in one eye from birth. He shoved his thick lenses up on his nose again with a grimy hand. "Floyd got his way last night, Mom.''

"The Bible,'' decided Mom firmly. She sat down in the rocker with the book in her lap. "We'll let Donald choose what story.''

"Aw gee, it's most always the Bible,'' began Floyd. But,

actually, none of us minded hearing Bible stories. Some of them had to do with giants, exciting battles, escapes, and other good stuff. Like Moses leading the people of Israel through the Red Sea with the Egyptians giving chase.

"I want to hear the one where the wicked Queen hammers the nail right through the general's head," I said. "Old what's-her-name."

"Jezebel. Well, all right." Mother licked her thumb and began to hunt through the heavy book on her lap.

In the green-gold light of dawn the following morning, I peeked through the crack beneath my window shade. There was Dad on his way to the barn to do the milking.

A little later, Mom cut my pancakes. She drizzled them with warm butter and syrup and replenished the supply for Floyd and Jack before she told us the news.

"Looks like we'll be moving soon. Your father got himself a new job."

Startled, the three of us gazed at him in silence when he came in and sat with thumbs hooked through the suspenders of his bib overalls. He rocked perilously back in his chair and laughed at our surprise.

"It's true," he admitted sheepishly. "When we move into Woonsocket, you'll be town kids. That'll probably take some getting used to."

Town boys! For my brothers it would mean the end of a special freedom. No more running wild. No more horseback riding unless they got invited to visit somebody else's farm. There would be boundaries.

But to me it opened up new vistas. A town would have a library with books to borrow. The streets would be lined with stores, and the glass windows of each store would be filled with things for a small boy to see when his father carried him down the main street.

There would be a school smelling of chalk and dust and paper and ink, a school larger than the building down the road from the farm.

40

During the past months, I'd picked up scraps of conversation with my name woven through them. "No way to educate a boy like our Don on a farm. . . ." "What Don needs is . . ." "Life in town would offer so much for Don as he grows older. . . ."

My brothers and I were full of questions. "Can we take the dog?" "What about the cattle?" "What about John, our hired man?" "How soon will it be?" "When can we start packing?"

"Sure we'll take the dog along," answered Mom, her whole face alight with smiles. "But John'll stay here to work for whatever family rents this farm. We'll not move till October, so that gives us a little time to plan. We'll pack some stuff with us and sell the rest."

She looked out the window at the parched fields and added, "A town'll feel good. Shops close at hand, and church right handy. The drought won't matter any more."

Dad looked the happiest I'd seen him look in ages. His old, jaunty air was back. He whacked his hat so hard against the edge of the table it raised a cloud of dust, and then he said teasingly, "Bet you boys'll never guess in a million years what I'm gonna do."

We thought and thought. Not one of us could picture him as anything but a dirt farmer in overalls with his felt hat pushed back on his head.

"Give up?" he prodded. "I'm a salesman, that's what I am!" He slapped his leg, roaring at our astonishment.

"What do . . . what're you gonna sell?"

"All kinds of things. It's called the Watkins Products line. You know the man who comes around every month or so and bamboozles your mother into ordering pepper and cake vanilla?"

Indeed we did. Especially me. I'd been housebound for so long that, like other visitors, the Watkins man had provided me a much-needed link with the outside world.

I laughed at the thought of my own father being an important person, carrying a suitcase of cans and bottles, and a pad of yellow order slips, and a pencil behind his ear.

He'd go around ringing doorbells and asking, "What'll you

41

have today, Madam?'' He'd come home each night with pockets jingling with quarters and nickels and dimes. When Mom wanted a new coat, he'd merely pull a few bills off the fat green roll in his back pocket and say, ''Here, Missus. And while you're at it, might as well pick out a coupla pairs of shoes.''

Folks depended upon mail order catalogs and door-to-door salesmen to bring them items not carried by the small town general stores. And so Dad would probably do pretty well.

Who could blame him for being lured into leaving a drought-sickened land and taking a job where the income did not depend on the capricious weather? I'm not sure he realized, at first, the cost of surrendering a familiar way of life.

He was a farmer through and through. He knew the soil and had worked hard, long hours. He'd developed a sense of pride in his crops and cattle. Out under the open sky, he could be himself. That was important to my father.

Now he would have to put on a mask. Floyd, being older than Jack and me, saw that. He made us laugh by pretending to be Dad when the grown-ups weren't around.

He flung open an imaginary bag full of enticing wares and said briskly: ''What'll it be today, lady? Just wait till I find the place in this gol darn catalog I have here. . . . Son of a bitch, here it is. . . . Lookee . . . any herb or spice you can think of right before your eyes!''

Dad wouldn't be able to talk like that in front of his customers.

Not long after breaking his momentous news, Dad drove to Woonsocket to look for a house. He found one with the necessary requirements, a couple of ground floor bedrooms, one for himself and Mom and another for me. The upstairs part of the house where Floyd and Jack were to sleep would have to remain a mystery to me. I had no back muscles. Although I weighed little, I was too floppy and unwieldy to carry up a steep staircase for the sake of satisfying my curiosity.

One thing I noticed right away. The new house had a flush

toilet with a roll of real, honest-to-goodness toilet paper instead of the Montgomery Ward catalog we'd used in the three holer on the farm. The family left off lingering in the bathroom. This one did not inspire the pleasant camaraderie of the outside privy. Worse than that, it seemed positively boring. Nobody ever held up the rest of the family by perusing the toilet paper before putting it to its proper use.

For a boy forced to remain in one of two positions, on his back or his stomach, a new house provided variety. Unfamiliar furniture joined the familiar. Tables, chairs, beds found at auctions or secondhand shops. I had a different window now, a different view. Instead of a rooster awakening me each morning, the rasping bell of Dad's Big Ben alarm clock intruded into my dreams.

People wandered in and out of the house to get acquainted. It didn't take Mom long to acquire a new set of coffee klatch friends. They brought me books, homemade donuts, other things. Again, I learned quickly to distinguish morbid curiosity seekers, the "poor Donnie" visitors from the sincere.

When my brothers' school chums dropped by, they usually hung around the couch and kept me company for a little while. I'd grown old enough, too, to be included in their games whenever it was possible.

Most exciting to me were the bags and boxes of stuff my father sorted on the floor where I could watch. Sometimes he unscrewed the cover of a particular bottle and gave me a whiff.

"Smell this perfume, Don, and tell me your opinion. Is it something the Missus might like for her birthday?"

Watkins was a big line. Dad carried every spice or herb or extract you could name . . . celery seed, garlic salt, oregano, thyme, ginger, clove, sweet basil, cinnamon, poultry seasoning, vanilla extract, maple or lemon extract, peppermint oil, cream of tartar, baking powder, and many other kitchen accoutrements.

He carried cleaners too, soaps, floor wax, furniture polish, and a strong pine oil for which Watkins was famous.

He carried a line of cosmetics and deodorants, shaving cream, talcum powder, both coconut oil shampoo and plain shampoo. The latter was an intriguing jellylike substance, blue in color. I begged Mom to try it on my own hair. He carried Soothie for sunburns, and toothpaste, and mouthwash guaranteed to cure bad breath.

An important part of his line were the patent medicines. Here he had to compete with the local drugstore. But Watkins' reputation was superb. Many people swore by their acid indigestion tonic, their famous petro-carbo salve, and their beef, iron and wine tonic, a pleasant-tasting appetite stimulant.

During this time, my parents kept hoping I would grow stronger, even that I would some day magically walk again. They knew the disease had either destroyed or damaged the motor nerves to some extent. But perhaps muscles could be reeducated.

Mom heard about a fortune-teller. Without saying a word to the family, she took off to consult with this psychic.

At supper she shared some startling information.

"Don't know how the fortune-teller did it. She's never seen me before in her life. But right out of the blue she says, 'You're having trouble with a sick boy at home.' "

"What else did she tell you?" demanded Dad.

"Well," Mom went on in a thoughtful voice, "she told me to rub Don's entire body with salad oil every single night. It's worth a try, don't you think, Kirk?"

"Can't hurt him any."

Every night after that, I was carried to the kitchen table and given a thorough rubdown with salad oil.

Mom felt pleased with the results. "What did I tell you, Kirk?" she exclaimed with a triumphant look in her eye. "It is helping! He's really picking up strength, don't you think?"

Another thing happened. A neighbor, Mrs. Sanborn, dropped by for coffee and said casually, "Why don't you take your boy to the bonesetters, Sue? They work wonders, those men do."

I listened intently to the conversation over the clinking of coffee cups. "You know Elsie Peterson's big girl? I mean the one who fell out of the haymow? She was real crazy till her Ma got the bonesetters to work on her. Yelled around kind of wildlike. The minute they pulled her back, something snapped into place. And there she was, calm and natural.''

"You sure the bonesetters did it?'' Mom looked doubtful. ''Mebbe the girl would've got better if her folks had just let her be.''

"It was the bonesetters all right,'' insisted Mrs. Sanborn. She pursed her lips in a knowing way. ''They proved it, too. Why one of 'em snapped her back out of place and there she was, all over again, babblin' and crazy in the head until they took pity and fixed her up. Didn't take them five minutes to get her in order.''

"I think I *will* take our Don,'' said Mom. ''I'll talk to Kirk about it tonight and see what he says.''

A shiver of excitement raced up and down my back.

On a school morning, after my brothers had left the house, Mom whipped through her household chores with unusual speed.

"Today we're going to the bonesetters' house,'' she announced with a lilt in her voice. She combed her hair and took off her apron, smoothing the wrinkles in her cotton dress as she did so.

She had no driver's license. That didn't matter though. South Dakota was so rural people didn't need a license to drive. Dad must have agreed to peddle his wares in town today. Mysteriously, the car was parked outside our house at ten in the morning.

"I understand they have such a mob that folks have to spend the night. I told your Dad I'd leave dinner in the pantry. I've packed a picnic for you and me.''

She hurried out to fix the back seat of the car with pillows for me to lie on. The bonesetters lived in a farmhouse several miles from town. We'd be going over stretches of bumpy dirt roads. I would doubtless feel every bump we hit since I had little flesh to pad my body.

As soon as the car was arranged to Mom's satisfaction, she came back to get me.

45

All during the ride I asked questions. "What will they do to me, Mom? Will it hurt? How long will it take?"

She could give me no answers.

Above the putter of the motor, I heard the clear song of a meadowlark. Mom pointed out her open window to the feathered creature perched jauntily on a fence post.

"See his black bib, Don? And how clear his song is!" She hesitated a moment, then added thoughtfully, "Better not count on walking out of there. It may take a long time to build up strength in your muscles. But God works in mysterious ways. If we have faith I'm sure He'll help. . . ."

"If we have faith . . ." When *she* said it, it sounded sincere. With Mom, it wasn't a religious garb like the one Preacher Hagglethorpe put on whenever he faced a parishioner. The tone of her voice didn't change. Her words were unsentimental, matter-of-fact.

She believed what she said. And somehow she'd got me to believing it too.

We'd read stories other than the gory ones about Jezebel and about David beaning Goliath, from the Bible. Quite often we read the kind that said "Ask and ye shall receive . . . Knock and it shall be opened unto you . . . If ye ask for bread, shall your Father give you a stone . . ."

The meanings were too deep for me. But my family's God was a God who could change things. Once, on the farm, I had heard Mom pray for rain. The next day brought a shower! And, too, all the time she was praying for me to get better, it was happening. Little by little.

So I was excited about going to the bonesetters.

"This isn't free, you know," remarked Mom presently. "Each family has to pay whatever they're able. But still, I feel certain the Almighty must be behind what they do. How else could they work such miracles? You heard the ladies tell about the girl who was out of her head."

46

"They said it took two men to hold her." I didn't dare ask the question that had bothered me ever since I heard that story. How could someone "go out of his head?" Was that where the real me lived, inside my head? And, if I went out of my head, where would I be? Who would be left inside the empty head to talk and hear and see?

It was a troubling matter. I could not get it into words.

"Mom, how did the bonesetters cure her? It didn't take her much time to get better, did it?"

"I guess each case is different," my mother said firmly. Meaning she didn't know the answer. "Well, this must be the place. Let's go in and see how they do it for ourselves. Mercy, look at the cars!"

To my surprise, the bonesetters' house resembled all the other farmhouses I'd ever seen, white, with a windbreak of poplars marching single file along one side, and a big red barn and a windmill out back. Serene cattle grazed in the fields, far enough away to look more like black splotches of ink spilled on the papery brown land.

In a pen, somewhere out of sight, a pig grunted. As Mom lifted me from the back seat of the car, a goat quit nibbling dried grass to stare with inquisitive eyes.

Cars lined the long dirt drive to the house. Many cars had simply pulled onto the parched grass to park, leaving room for others to move in and out. People drifted to and from the house, some with crutches or canes, others looking perfectly healthy.

Nobody seemed to be using the brass knocker, so Mom pushed the door open with an elbow and, with me yet in her arms, sat down in one of the chairs in the hall.

It was crowded there, old men, children, babies, mothers, young girls in their teens, boys in patched jeans and some with better clothes, farmers, businessmen.

The man sitting next to us on one side had a crutch, and I saw two wheelchairs, one holding a man in flannel pajamas.

In the other wheelchair, a girl was strapped. I saw she had to be restrained that way because her whole body shook and trembled.

The wheelchairs were in a sitting room adjacent to the hall. That room, too, had lots of people in it. Two or three grown-ups were lying on the floor with coats tucked around them.

"Try not to stare," whispered Mom.

Fascinated, I soon discovered ways to look at my surroundings without seeming to stare.

The door at the end of the hall must lead into the clinic. While I watched, it swung open. Out came an older boy with a twisted foot, and after him, his father, a thin, worried-looking man with dirty fingernails and a shirt unbuttoned at the collar. The boy limped. It was impossible to guess if either of them felt any different because of the bonesetters.

A mother took her baby inside next, bundled so carefully into a pink blanket nobody could see how sick it was, or how deformed.

One or two people looked so healthy I asked in a low voice, "But why are they here? What's wrong with them?"

"We'll talk about it later," Mom whispered back.

A lady with twin boys my age opened her purse and took out two lollipops for them. To my astonishment, suddenly she clicked her purse open once again and produced a third lollipop for me! She smiled and handed it to Mom.

With a swift glance, she looked my way and turned and asked Mom, "How old is he?"

Mom had torn the paper off the candy and put it in my mouth. I felt pleased to think she would relax her rule about accepting candy from strangers. Eagerly I sucked the orange lollipop, trying to enjoy as much of it as possible, lest she change her mind.

In an instant it came to me that this lady thought I had remained in some sort of baby stage, unable to answer questions for myself. She thought I was different from other children! I was humiliated but only for a moment. I set her straight by answering her question myself. "I'm six. How old are your little boys?"

I very much wanted to know what was wrong with them. Other than appearing as fragile as the fine china plates Mom stored in a cupboard until Thanksgiving time, I saw no hint of sickness.

Their mother anticipated my question. "My boys were born with a curvature of the spine. It doesn't show much now, but it will as soon as they grow, if nothing is done to correct it."

I licked my lollipop in silence, letting the delicious orange juice trickle down the back of my tongue while Mom explained about my siege with polio.

Enough people had moved in and out to leave a small couch vacant. She plumped the cushions a bit and set me down. One of the twins came over and squatted on the floor to talk. "Where do you live? What do you like to do best?"

We chattered back and forth, paying no mind to the two mothers who were busy sharing notes on their children's ailments.

Throughout the day people streamed in and out of the clinic. One of the bonesetters came to the door occasionally and greeted a few patients as if they were old acquaintances.

I looked at him curiously, a simple stocky farmer of Scandinavian background, dressed in bib overalls, very tall. His face was sunburned. I could see the white line across his forehead where his hat sat whenever he went outside to work in the fields.

When the other bonesetter came to the door, there was nothing unusual about him either. He seemed younger, taller, more sunburned. If these plain men could heal people, why couldn't my mother do it? Or Grandpa Merritt? Or anyone else?

"It's a gift," Mom told me patiently when I asked a second time. "I told you that, Donald. It's a God-given gift. Some people have it, some don't."

Mom liked to be around people. She made friends easily. By nightfall she had several new acquaintances. One family offered to trade two pieces of fried chicken for a pint of our good farm milk to feed their baby.

There had not been enough hours in the day for the bonesetters to see every person who had come. The ones left ate their picnic suppers and figured out ways to spend the night. Some went back to their cars to have some privacy. Others, like Mom and me, curled up on couches or on the floor, using coats for blankets and pillows.

My turn to see the bonesetters came early the next morning. The twins were sound asleep on the floor, their mother on a couch beside them. A few people were quietly eating cold breakfast donuts, hardboiled eggs, oranges and such, and sipping coffee from thermos bottle cups.

Mom carried me into the clinic. The older bonesetter took me into his strong arms and set me on a table covered with padding.

"So you're Donald. Hello."

He turned to Mom. "Please remove the boy's shirt and loosen his trousers so I can have a look."

When he bent to probe my back with strong, sure fingers, I could see the dust on his work shoes. The mixture of barn-and-earth odors clinging to his clothes was as familiar to me as the smell of his clean old clothes. I felt completely at ease.

For a while he felt up and down my spine from neck to seat. He pulled my legs and aligned my body to his satisfaction, then went on pressing, pulling, probing for what seemed like a long time.

In the silence a fly buzzed. Through the open window I heard the billy goat split the autumn air with a sorrowful bleat.

At last the bonesetter rubbed a finger over my thin ribs. "Got to get some meat on you, Don. Eat a little more, hear? Next time you come, I want to see a few extry pounds on you."

Bring him back for more treatments," he told my mother. "We'll have this fellow sitting up before long."

"Thank you." Mom handed him a folded bill from her purse.

And so we started home, bearing inside ourselves the mystery of what happened with very plain people inside a very plain farmhouse. Who were the bonesetters? They had mumbled no

50

incantations or prayers. They had not discussed religion with any of those patients who waited long hours in their office. They had received no special training, such as chiropractors do, before embarking upon this work of theirs. How had they discovered their power to heal?

We were to visit them several times more. Each time we waited, we listened to conversations relating the miraculous things they had done.

Sometimes one of the farmers worked on me, sometimes the other. When I first went to the bonesetters' place, my head lolled forward on my chest whenever any adult held me in an upright position. Gradually those firm, massaging hands strengthened long unused muscles. And of course the nightly rubdowns at home helped to continue the healing process.

The bonesetter's prediction came true. By the end of October I was able to sit up without another person helping to support me. A major victory! The entire world, indoors and out, looks different when one is able to view it sitting up. One has a little bit of a hold on it.

One is not so helpless.

To celebrate, Dad and Mom connived together and bought me a gift at one of Grandfather Merritt's auctions, a roomy wicker baby stroller. At six, I didn't give a darn that such a conveyance was ordinarily reserved for infants. I was pleased as punch.

Now Mom could push me up and down the sidewalks in town, into stores and out. With another person's assistance, I had become mobile!

"When we want to go anyplace I can take you in your chariot," laughed Mom.

"I can go to the fireworks next Fourth of July," I planned out loud when she was wheeling me down the main street of town one day. "And the circus. Dicky Sanborn told me it comes to town every year when school lets out."

"We'll see. Right now let's settle for Sam Warner's soda fountain. I've got enough nickels for an ice cream cone a piece.

There's a lot else to think about besides circuses and fireworks.''

I could tell she had something on her mind. Later in the afternoon when she was rolling out biscuits for supper, it came out of its own accord:

"Your Dad and I been talking, Don.'' She laid the floury rolling pin on the table and came over and sat down. "We've heard about a big childrens' hospital in Glasgow, Minnesota. Maybe if we could take you there, a doctor could do something for you. A large hospital knows all the new treatments.''

My heart drummed.

"Could they get me to walk again?'' I asked after a while.

"I hope so. You understand we'd have to leave you there for a long time, Donald. But we could write letters. And your Uncle Harry and Aunt Maud would be able to visit you on Sundays.''

Her eyes misted. "It'd be worth anything in the whole world if you could walk again.''

That very night I dreamed I was playing Hide and Seek with Floyd and Jack and Paul Peterson and the twins.

"You're it, you're it!'' shouted Floyd. So I hid my eyes against the side of the barn and counted the only way I knew, by tens to one hundred. The darkening sky was streaked with the wild pink banners of a fading sunset, and shadows moved across the land.

As soon as I reached one hundred, I pivoted on one foot and began to run.

*four*

---

OUR family never made a to-do over important matters. At the end of January, when I'd been housebound by winter weather for a long time, Dad bundled me up and took me out on his delivery rounds.

He left me outside in the car in a nest of blankets while he took his products up to each house. I was glad to be outside. All along the way, I drew deep breaths and pretended I was a dragon with smoke billowing out of my mouth. Dad entertained me by running through his repertoire of stories about his bachelor days in the Canadian woods. He always spiced up the same old stories with new details to make them interesting.

We made numerous stops. By dusk, the paper sacks in the back of the car had dwindled until only two were left.

"Both of these go to old Missus Flack over on 9th. Then we better get home to supper, eh Don?"

His supply of stories had petered out. On the way home, Dad fell strangely quiet, clearing his throat a time or two as if he wanted to speak but could not. As he carried me into the house, blankets and all, he said abruptly,

"The letter from Glascow came yesterday. The hospital has room for you. I guess the Missus'll be taking you on the train next week."

No fanfare. No special preparations. Mom washed and ironed my Sunday best, and set about preparing pans of fried pheasant and loaves of homemade bread to leave Dad and Floyd and Jack the week she'd be away.

Since I was unable to cope with such an enormous change before it happened, I put thoughts of the hospital out of my head. I had the train trip to think about, anyhow. That in itself would be fun. Few boys from Woonsocket, South Dakota, had ever been lucky enough to ride on a train for any distance. I found I was the envy of the neighborhood.

The news spread. Young visitors popped in and out of our house to check things for themselves.

"You lucky bum! Spending a night on a train!"

"My Pa's been on one. He says some of 'em can go seventy-five miles an hour!"

"Git the porter to lift you into the top berth," suggested one enterprising young friend. "Your Ma's pretty heavy. Probably she'd rather take the low one anyhow."

I had not thought about it. It sounded like a fine idea.

"Wisht it was me. I'd like to miss school."

"How soon'll you be coming back?"

"What're they gonna do to you, Don?"

I had to admit I didn't know. But I bristled with importance. I was going on a train, wasn't I? And a lot of my friends wished they could trade places and be me.

When we lived on the farm, one of the highlights of the day had been to get to see the train whizz by on the tracks a few miles from home. It slowed down at the Cuthbert platform only long enough for a trainman to reach out deftly with a long metal hook, and grab the mailbag hanging on a post near the tracks.

Other than that, the train never stopped unless a passenger needed to get off or on.

Woonsocket was different. The passenger train did stop at the Woonsocket station every evening, a noisy black monster belching clouds of smoke.

The night Dad lifted me onto it and checked Mom's tickets while she got settled in a red plush seat, the roaring in my ears matched the noise of the train getting ready to depart.

I could hardly say goodbye. This was not a picture in a storybook. This was me, Donald Kirkendall, leaving home to go to a strange city!

Various thoughts might be racing through Mom's head too, but, on the outside at least, she kept her composure.

The train chugged underway. After the conductor came by to punch our tickets, Mom produced supper from one of the two shoeboxes my father had stored beneath our seats.

There were bologna sandwiches with slices of dill pickle. There were American cheese sandwiches, and cookies, and hard-boiled eggs with an ample supply of salt folded into a scrap of oiled paper.

For a special treat, she took two dimes from her purse and bought bottles of orange soda pop for us both when the man came through the cars selling it.

After we'd finished the last crumb of supper, she said, "I brought the copy of *Lassie Come Home*. Would you like to hear a chapter?"

"Gee . . . no thanks." I was finding too much to see when the train pulled in and out of stations to concentrate on a story. At the very next stop, a man with a waxed moustache and shiny shoes boarded the train. He walked down the aisle to our seat.

"I believe you are occupying my place, Madam," he told Mom.

"You are right." To my amazement, Mom laughed. "My son, Don, here, has the bottom berth. I have the bottom berth across the aisle. I was just keeping him company."

Quickly she gathered her belongings and moved across the aisle. "We can chat from our two aisle seats real comfortably," she remarked. "Besides, the porter will be by soon to make our beds."

I wasn't too disappointed about the top berth being occupied. It turned out to be intriguing enough to go to sleep in the curtained lower berth with its handy shelf above my pillow.

"I'll leave your window shade partway up, like this," said Mom. "You can look out at the scenery for a while. Don, if you need anything, you can reach the bell with your left hand, can't you?"

I tried and nodded.

"Good night."

"Good night."

For a long time I watched the shadowy forms of houses, trees, bushes, fences fly by. At last the haunting whistle of the speeding train lulled me to sleep.


Once I reached my destination, my transformation was shockingly sudden. Unasked for. Unexpected.

The three-day stint on the isolation ward was bad enough. But it was more difficult by far, when I awakened on the Small Boys Ward with the ego-smashing sensation I had become a blob.

Mom was on her way back to South Dakota. I was no longer important to anyone.

The boys looked me over and plied me with questions. Overcome with homesickness and fright, I could not answer. I turned my face to the wall.

Gradually, I began to drink in the details of my new surroundings. Almost at once, I noticed how a few lucky children were more mobile than others. It soon became apparent, though, that the strict rules of the hospital sentenced them to spend most of the day in bed like everyone else.

When the nurses were in good humor we could holler back and forth to each other.

I began to get acquainted with Ted, the small blond boy in the bed adjacent to mine. But in two days he went home. I missed him sorely. He'd been a jolly neighbor, lifting my spirits with his wisecracks.

"Never mind," consoled the nurse who found me staring disconsolately at the vacated bed. "In a day or so you'll have a new boy there to talk to."

My new neighbor turned out to be a boy much sicker than any of the rest of us. His mother, a silent woman, had bloodshot eyes from weeping.

"We'll get him into a single room as soon as possible," the head nurse told her. "This is only a temporary arrangement."

A whisper passed up and down the ward. "That's Johnny Vanessa. He's been here before. I heard doc say they can't help him none. His bones are rotting."

Horrified, I tried to blot the picture out of my mind. It kept coming back, that sickening vision of rotting bones.

I woke in the morning relieved to find the bed empty.

"Did he . . . did he go home?"

"Naw. He died. In the middle of the night while you were sleeping. You missed it," piped up a kid on the other side of the ward.

Was he teasing? Jolted, I looked to see. But no, he was merely giving me a realistic answer.

Things like that happened on the ward.

Daily, I watched other boys get wheeled off to surgery. I saw them return, silent forms, swathed in bandages, on the long stretchers. I knew, with dread, my turn would come. But when?

The hospital staff held to one particularly odd rule. The half hour from seven until seven-thirty each night was a time of production. Every young patient on every one of the three wards must learn to keep to the required schedule. This was grunting time, the time of the day we were, in uncouth terms, required "to do our number two."

The stench of fifty children simultaneously filling their bedpans was unbearable. I never did get used to it. But the consequence of refusing to do so, deliberately or unintentionally, was worse.

Our tormentors allowed us to miss one day in the rigid schedule. Woe to the constipated lad who missed twice in a row. The following Tuesday night, instead of chuckling over a Charlie Chaplin movie, the offender would find himself banished, bed and all, to the large ugly main bathroom down the hall. Here he must remain for the duration of the show.

The Tuesday night movie was one of the few regular diversions provided by the hospital. The nurses had custody of the few toys given to the hospital. They were stingy about loaning out these items. They were "good toys" and nobody wanted to see them get messed up. Adults understood this logic, but not the children who pined for playthings.

So, by the time Tuesday evening rolled around, we were delighted at the prospect of bona fide entertainment. Nobody dared complain if it was our ward's night to view the movie backward. The nurse in charge never took time to show the movie twice. Instead, one ward's beds were rolled around in front of the screen. The other ward was relegated to the back side where they saw the picture and captions through the screen, backward.

One morning, in place of my breakfast tray, I found a sugar candy treat. I regarded it with mixed feelings. Today must be my day for surgery.

The doctors were going to fix me up! I'd been told they would put me to sleep while they did it. I wanted to be fixed, but, still, I was worried. With my own eyes I'd witnessed stretchers come and go.

I had seen the bodies swathed in bandages.

Well, I could endure a few bandages in order to walk again. This time, I felt certain I would walk. Mom had prayed about the matter for a long time. And I had muttered my own prayers too, with childish faith.

The great room where I was wheeled on the stretcher had

glaring lights. Dismayed, I took in the doctors with gauze masks hanging around their necks, the stethoscopes, the bottles of antiseptic, the bandages, the tweezers and tubes lying ready and waiting, and the row of mean-looking surgical knives.

"Are you . . . gonna *cut* . . . me?"

"Oh no," a doctor assured me, winking at the others. "No cutting. We're going to fix you up, young man. That's what you want us to do, don't you?"

The ether cone was over my nose before I could give him an answer. A voice behind the stretcher said, "Be a good boy and help us count to one hundred."

Drowsily I began . . . one . . . two . . . three . . . four . . . I was falling and could not catch myself . . . falling . . . falling . . .

Hours later I opened my eyes on the ward and immediately got sick to my stomach.

"Mom! Oh Mom!"

A nurse held the basin steady while I retched again. "Your mother is in South Dakota, Don. But your Uncle Harry called. He'll be around to scc you on Sunday afternoon. He wanted to know how you were and I told him fine."

Even in that groggy state, a thrill went through me.

I was fine! Did I have a straight, good usable pair of legs, then?

"How's my legs?" I mumbled. "Oh . . . oh . . . basin, quick!"

"You won't be using your legs for a while," she told me when I was done. "Can't you tell? You're in a body cast from your neck to your toes."

Her rubber soles squeaked as she went over to rinse the basin at the sink. When she returned, she added, "Don't worry, there's a hole cut out of the front and back of the cast so you can go to the bathroom. And your arms are free."

"I gotta go now," I said.

Briskly, she opened the door of my bedstand. "Uh-oh, your urinal is gone. I'm going off duty but I'll tell someone to bring you a clean one."

Must be night time. Groggily, I noticed the lights of the ward were off. The room was quiet.

Now I was getting desperate to relieve myself but nobody came. The spell of ether was upon me. Hard to tell if I was awake or asleep. And so sick! Oh . . . oh. I moaned in the dark.

"I can't reach my bell! Hurry! Please!"

A light snapped on. Miss Blood, the head nurse, the one I despised was at my side. Hatchet-faced. Never a smile.

"For pity sakes, stop shouting like that. I was busy and came as fast as I could."

Angrily, she shoved the urinal against my cast. It was an unfamiliar feeling. I was too sick and too desperate to aim properly.

A jet of urine hit her square in the eye.

Wham-bang! Wham-bang! What was happening?

That infuriated nurse was slapping the face of a small boy just down from surgery, encased in a body cast and only half conscious. Wham-bang, wham-bang, wham-bang.

"That should teach you!" she stormed. "Wait until the supervisor hears this!"

For the rest of my hospital stay, a full six months, I was incontinent.

"Don't feel bad about wetting the bed," a young nurse comforted me time and again. "It's because you're sick. You'll get over it."

Some day I would. Maybe at home when Mom could lift me in and out of the bathroom. Right now I felt far too frightened to make any further attempt to use a bedpan or urinal.

Days passed. I yearned to ask one of the doctors about my legs. They seemed engrossed in the deformity or handicap apart from the child. Many of them found it difficult to treat a patient as a person possessing real feelings.

60

Several doctors did not care if you had pain. One day I overheard a doctor say to a nurse, "Let the kid alone. Nobody ever died of pain, you know."

I had seen that very doctor take a tiny two-year-old's foot in his hands and snap it with a sickening crunch to straighten it before he put on a cast. No anesthetic.

At the time I could do nothing but pull my cover over my head with my one good hand to drown out the baby's screams.

"Why did he hurt him that way?" I whispered to the nurse who brought my lunch tray.

"The bone hadn't set properly so he had to break it and start over again," she told me. "That's all."

Later I would have some of that cold-blooded cruelty practiced on myself. My body grew stiff from being encased in the cast. To break the adhesions, which formed during that time, my doctor simply removed the cast and raised me to a sitting position. Without warning, he let me fall back on the bed again.

He paid not the slightest heed to the blood-curdling screams of pain, but continued to do this over and over while the boys in the surrounding beds gaped, intrigued by such a show.

Long before that happened, I had watched for one of the friendlier doctors to come by my bed. When he did, I ventured to ask, "How'm I doing, doc? How soon'll I walk?"

Puzzled, he looked down at me. "Walk? Your cast will be on for a few more months. Then we'll have to see. No doubt you'll be able to move about some with back and leg braces."

The glorious picture faded from my head, that picture of myself tearing through the backyards of Woonsocket in games of Tag, Hide and Seek, Cops and Robbers, Prisoner's Base, Cowboys and Indians.

With the click of the fingers, it was gone.

God! I hate you, hear? I'm not gonna talk to you any more, God. I asked you and asked you.

But later on I determined I would pray more and ask again. I wanted to walk like other boys.

61

Nobody had bothered to tell me the truth. The doctors had made an irrevocable decision. In order to prevent my legs from curling up in a grotesque fashion as my body matured, they had severed the cords. They were correct in saying I might reach a stage when I would be able to propel myself in tortuous ways with a heavy steel brace and crutches. But by now they were already certain of one thing: I would never move freely, normally, with ease again.

In the regimented, Victorian hospital, days passed heavily, without end. Where now was the other Don, the one who had been pushed like a king up and down the streets of Woonsocket in his wicker buggy, oh sweet chariot! Where was the small boy bundled into mittens and hat and blankets, the one who rode across the snow in his Grandfather's cutter, or on the Watkins route in his father's car?

What had happened to the child who sat propped in a chair at the kitchen table, practicing a left-handed alphabet while his mother fried sweet-smelling pieces of pheasant and potatoes and gravy for dinner?

Without play, our life in the hospital became unbearable. We invented our own amusements. Perhaps the doctors and nurses charted us simply as cases of osteomyelitus or TB of the bone, or congenital defect, or polio. But we were, indeed, a ward full of boys with hearts and minds of our own.

One boy, Charlie Staffenhauser, baffled every nurse in the place by turning up in a bed at the opposite end of the ward. How did he manage it, encased in a body cast covering everything except one leg? Simple . . . he "walked" from bed to bed on his hands.

A great pleasure was to tease the janitor, a morose Armenian fellow who spoke broken English. His name was Carl.

Carl hated children. Why, then, did he choose to work in this hospital? It didn't make sense. Each day, bound by duty, he cleaned the main part of the ward and then proceeded to go from

62

one bed to the next, swishing his big mop beneath the furniture along the way.

Each day the stronger, bolder boys pulled the same trick. As soon as Carl hunched over to mop beneath a bed, the boy in the one behind him grabbed the end of his mop handle.

A tug of war began. Carl uttered a fierce growl and yanked for all he was worth. The boy on the opposite end yanked too, and imitated the growl. The game continued until at last the poor janitor reached a point of explosion.

"You . . . you . . . you . . . *bad boy*! Stop zat, I tell you!"

He realized it was out of the question to lay a hand on a culprit. A nurse might have this privilege, not a janitor. So he was forced to limit his anger to expletives instead of action.

He threatened, though. "Stop zat or I vill tell ze nurse!"

Whenever the boy on the handle end got tired of the joke he let go. Sometimes Carl lost his balance and sat down hard. But he never did report any of us to the nurse in charge. He may have thought a complaint would cost him his job. Or, perhaps he possessed a smidgeon of compassion after all.

A prank or two like that lightened our dullest days. But the person who did the most to raise me out of the doldrums was my Uncle Harry.

Visiting hours were scheduled on Sunday afternoon. You had to be on your deathbed before a visitor would be permitted "in" on any other day.

During my stay at the hospital, Uncle Harry only missed one Sunday. That was the day his sister died. He telephoned a message to me, a promise to make it the following Sunday afternoon.

Uncle Harry was married to my mother's sister, Maud. Proudly, I claimed him as *my* Uncle Harry. But, as soon as he hit the ward, it became obvious he was everybody else's Uncle Harry, too.

Uncle Harry was a Frenchman. Put together the facial characteristics, the receding hairline, the eyes, the chin of a short version

of General de Gaulle, and the debonair spirit of Maurice
Chevalier, and you might come close to someone a little like Uncle
Harry.

It takes a special person to visit a ward of sick, deformed
children. Aunt Maud couldn't take it. She stayed home and Uncle
Harry came alone.

He was a child at heart, a prankster and a clown. Somewhat
warily, he observed the strict outlook of the hospital staff. After
that he made an immediate and long-lasting decision to side with
the children.

Since he owned and supervised the operation of a large factory, Uncle Harry was a wealthy man. Each Sunday he arrived
bearing gifts, boxes of crayons, drawing paper, airplanes, cars,
storybooks, games, puzzles.

He did not give the impression of being in a hurry or having
other more important things to do. After a leisurely visit with me,
during which he could make me laugh so hard I felt I would break
my cast, he went from bed to bed and spent time with the other
boys.

I rested content with the new toy he had brought to me. When
giggles issued from other beds, I would confide proudly to the
new boy in the bed next to mine, "That's *my* Uncle Harry."

One of the best toys Uncle Harry brought me was a dump
truck, a sturdy one with battery operated headlights that flashed
on and off. I longed to be down on the floor so I could play
with it properly. But we soon thought of a way to put it to use.

As soon as the nurses' backs were turned at mealtimes, we
had a gentleman's agreement concerning the trading of food. The
system worked quite naturally, according to likes and dislikes. I
was practically the only boy who possessed an insatiable appetite
for cheese.

The day after the truck arrived was a cheese day.

"Hey, Donald, pass down your new truck and we'll load her
up," suggested an older boy at one end of the ward.

No sooner said than done. Before long the truck raced toward

64

my bed with a superb supply of cheese. My neighbor leaned out and swooped it off the floor and handed it to me.

I began eating. I ate and I ate and I ate. I ate some more. And I ate some more after that, too.

Only one piece left to go . . . and in walked a nurse. Now I was so full of cheese I felt as if I might throw up. I looked sideways at the last piece on my tray. I simply could not manage it. I had had enough!

The nurse lifted my tray and eyed the cheese grimly before she handed it back to me. "Young man, don't you know we eat everything on our plates at this hospital? Here, eat your cheese."

Slowly, I began to munch.

We thought up new games. After we'd driven the nurses out of their skulls by vocalizing, we resorted to moving whatever parts of our anatomy that were movable. We collected rubber bands and shot them at one another. Any exposed area of the human body was considered an acceptable target. Many boys became proficient at hitting the target.

Aside from my arms, I had the most enticing exposed area of anyone on the ward. My rear end. Wow! When I got hit dead on center, how it did sting!

I tried to remain under the covers when rubber bands were flying. One day when the resident doctor stopped by to examine my cast, he failed to pull the covers over me. There I was, on my stomach, seat available as a target. I was lost in the book Uncle Harry had brought me the previous Sunday. A barrage of rubber bands took me completely by surprise.

"Help! Help! Oh *stop*! For Pete's sake, stop!"

Four nurses rushed to the scene. But every rubber band had been whisked out of sight. Loyally I hid the few in my bed under the pillow.

"It's not fair," I complained to Uncle Harry next time he visited. "I got no way to protect myself. And I can't shoot rubber-bands with only one good hand."

That was true.

"What I need is a rubber band machine gun," I told him.

Uncle Harry's expression remained sober, considering the seriousness of the situation. But laughter flickered in his eyes.

"A rubber band machine gun?" he repeated. "Donald, you do beat all!"

The following Sunday afternoon he appeared with . . . . *a rubber band machine gun.*

"I hope you appreciate this, young fellow." He tried to keep a straight face as he handed it over. "I asked my secretary and several workers at the factory to do a little research on the subject. They combed the entire city before they found what you wanted."

"Golly, Uncle Harry! It's a real one? Oh, Golly!"

I hadn't known such an item existed. Had he found it or had he invented it? I could hardly wait to try it out.

"It'll take fifteen rubber bands at a clip," Uncle Harry informed me. "Can I try it out, or do you want to be the first?"

_five_

I had dreamed of stepping off the train in Woonsocket with a straight back and two legs that worked. Instead I arrived home encased in a steel and horsehide contraption. My brace covered both back and legs. It was heavy. It transformed me into a dead weight for anyone to carry. I faced another disappointment, too. Even this marvelous twentieth-century invention did not enable me to stand alone or move.

I had to be carried. Whenever I wanted to get dressed or undressed, take a bath or just go to the toilet, I needed the assistance of another person.

Mom tried her best to comfort. "Never mind, Donald. So you can't walk yet. Don't give up. Meantime, the brace will strengthen your muscles."

What muscles? I wanted to shout. I loathed the thing, but the doctor had said I must wear it and that was that. To my parents, a doctor's word was as good as the Lord's.

I had outgrown the buggy. For a year I went every place

in a red wagon, propped with plenty of pillows. And then I got my first wheelchair. I felt like I would burst with joy. No more lying down for most of the day . . . no more baby buggy or wagon! For hours and hours, if I wanted to, I could sit in my chair.

It was a three-wheeler, this chair of mine—two big wheels in front and a little one in back. When I sat in it, it was like being perched on top of a pinnacle. And, I soon found out, as precarious. It was an annoyingly unbalanced piece of equipment. It tipped at home or on the main street of town. Once or twice, it tipped in church, spilling me into the aisle. Right while Preacher Haggelthorpe was hollering at the top of his lungs.

One time he'd chosen a text from Obadiah. Something about God promising to destroy the sinful kingdom from the face of the earth. He'd worked himself into a case of laryngitis, practically, before he got around to informing his dear flock that they could be among the righteous who would be saved, when Otto Proudhammar, slouched in the pew directly ahead of me, let out a terrible snore. Old Otto's snores were worse than my father's farts, much worse. I snickered and Floyd kicked the wheel of my chair lightly, warning me to stop before Mom caught on . . . and over I went.

I broke a leg and an elbow in that chair but I didn't care. It was splendid to be mobile. Now, except for the long, inclement winter months when I had to spend most days indoors, I could be part of the gang and take part in their games, brace, chair, and all.

Farming was in Dad's blood. He didn't stay a Watkins man for long. He went back to the soil. We moved from small farm to small farm in the Woonsocket and Cuthbert area.

In the good years, we had fed buttermilk to the pigs and had sold our cream-rich milk in five-gallon cans. But even in the poorest years, the years of grasshoppers and dust, we managed to have enough.

Mom cried and cried when she could not afford a new winter

coat. It was humiliating to have to go to Ladies Guild in one that was ragged and darned. But still, there was food on the table. Never once did we go to bed without supper.

When we had eaten the last of our chickens, there was always plenty of pheasant. Nobody ever got tired of that. Succulent, meaty pieces of pheasant, fried crisp and served up with gravy and slices of homemade bread. Sometimes the game warden dropped by to take pot luck. He didn't bat an eye when he saw that heaping platter of pheasant coming to the table out of season. He ate as much of it as Dad and when he finally was stuffed, he coughed discreetly into his napkin and complimented my mother.

"That was mighty delicious chicken, Miz Kirkendall. Mighty delicious. As good as my wife Sally can cook, if I do say so myself."

"Thank you and come again, any time you're in the area." Mom couldn't help chuckling under her breath at the secret joke between them.

She was a good cook, the game warden was right about that. Our kitchen range had four plates on it. A reservoir at the back made it possible to have hot water at any time. There was an enormous oven, too. One day Mom heard about a friend on a neighboring farm who had typhoid. Early the next morning she got up and began baking bread. By nightfall she'd baked thirty-six loaves, enough for both the neighbor family and ourselves.

And what meals she set before the farm hands in summertime . . . memories of hospital fare, creamed asparagus and soggy potatoes, left me when I sniffed the smells coming out of my mother's kitchen.

The hospital was miles away. I was home safe. I was not a blob any more, an anonymous bunch of arms and legs in a doctor's hands. I was Donald Kirkendall. I was me, and I could do anything! Well, practically anything.

For one thing, I soon taught myself to read. In the blistering summer heat, my brace chafed something terrible. Going outside in the blazing sun would make me sweat more and of course then the brace would rub worse. Bored, I picked up one of Floyd's books about the Rover Boys.

"Can't you stop sewing for a while and read this to me?" I begged Mom.

She let her foot come up off the treadle for a minute. "I reckon you could do it yourself if you tried, Don. Let's see, why don't you begin by spelling out words to me while I hem my new apron. I was getting ready to set the cover on the machine anyway."

While she sewed, I spelled. An hour went by, then two. Excitement tingled down my spine. I was getting the hang of it! At last Mom rolled up her sewing. It was time to cook supper. A triumphant look passed between us.

"You *can* do it, Don. I knew you could!"

"I can read!" I gloated to everyone at the table that night. Over and over I said it. "I can read! I can read!" A new world opened itself to me that day. The chair had brought me one kind of mobility. Reading would bring another.

It dawned on me . . . books could carry me anywhere, no legs needed. I'd already gotten an inkling of it with Mom's night-time reading. But this was different. Now I could go into those distant lands myself, without a single person standing by to help.

"Son of a bitch!" exclaimed Dad when I stammered out a paragraph from the Rover Boys to demonstrate my new skill. "Mebbe in the fall we'll be able to get you back and forth to school, Don. It's about time, isn't it?"

I was enjoying every minute at home. I was growing much slower than other boys my age but finally I outgrew my cumbersome brace. It began to chafe worse than ever after it got too small. Before any adult mentioned it to me, I surmised I would soon have to take the night train north to the hospital in order to be fitted with a new brace. How I dreaded it!

This time the doctors discussed the possibility of more surgery. Now that I was eight, I was on the Middle Boys Ward, but I was young enough yet and naive enough to look for a miracle all over again. Why would they bother to operate, I reasoned to myself, unless they expected something to happen?

They had not told me they were only planning to break the adhesions beginning to form between the severed cords in my legs.

"This time I'll walk for sure, Dr. Williams. I will, won't I?"

"I hope so."

The liar! He knew it was impossible but lacked the guts to help me face the truth. Besides that, he was a busy man.

Unexpectedly, before I got out of the isolation room, onto the Middle Boys Ward, I gained a little power.

The nurse who lifted me from wheelchair to bed sized me up and decided a boy my age was too old for bedsides. She set me on the bed, pulled up the covers, and left the room, closing the door behind her.

I found myself in one of those high, narrow hospital beds with my bell, as usual, just out of reach. I could not press it even with the tips of my good fingers.

Lucky I didn't have to go. Not yet. But golly I was getting thirstier by the minute. With my door slammed shut I could barely hear the voices of kids calling back and forth on the ward. I couldn't hear a nurse chatting to a doctor as they went by, although I did catch a fleeting glimpse of a starched white cap and a bald head through the glass window at the top of the door.

My tongue grew uncomfortably dry. The roof of my mouth prickled. And the tantalizing, cool, clear jug of water sat on my bedstand with a glass straw stuck into its top.

To heck with the nurses. I could get my own water. With my good hand I clung to the edge of the mattress and inched my way toward the water jug. Ah . . . now! Glowing with triumph at finding myself sufficient, I reached.

The crash of a body from high bed to floor, plus the terrified screams that followed, pierced the walls of the isolation unit. The door flew open and I was surrounded by aghast adults.

Lucky me. This happened to be the very day of the week the doctors were on hand to make their rounds. Terror gave way to victory. It took only a split second for me to realize what a profound effect my bellows had produced. Promptly, I scrunched my eyelids shut and shrieked again for all I was worth.

Between yells I took a peek and was delighted to see an irate doctor taking the head nurse to task. In fact, it looked as if every one of those nurses would get a thorough dressing down right in front of me!

"Idiots!" shouted one M.D. "I'd think anybody would know better than to go off and leave a kid in that condition without a restraint or bedsides. He cast a withering glance at one of the poor nurses who trembled and turned away.

An orthopedic specialist shook his head. "If I ever hear of a case like this again . . . I'll take action. Believe me, I'll take action! Every one of you nurses is responsible to see to it nothing happens to this boy. Give him the best care possible. And . . ." he looked back over his shoulder and thundered, "for God's sake, pay attention to what you're doing from now on. Did anyone stop to think about the hospital's reputation?"

For a solid week I was the king. I accepted the role and played it to the hilt. The call bell was set within easy reach and I took great pleasure in ringing it many times a day. One flick of my little finger brought a nurse to my side. I was Aladdin rubbing his magic lamp and having a geni appear!

After a while things settled back to normal and I became just one of the kids on the Middle Boys Ward. One day I was wheeled up to surgery. Hours later I returned under the familiar, sickening spell of ether. Encased, too, in the same old body cast as before . . . head to toe.

Dare I inquire about walking now?

I waited. Months later when my cast was being sawed off, the question remained on the tip of my tongue. I was in the emergency room. Out of the corner of my eye, I could see a new and larger two-legged brace propped against the wall waiting for me.

72

Inside me was a well of unshed tears. I refused to let the doctors see me cry.

Oh God, I asked you again and you didn't hear. God Almighty, if you're so smart, why can't you get me to walk?

God . . . where are you now?

Dreary day after dreary day passed by. I wanted to be home and I thought that spring would never come. Uncle Harry's visits helped some but toward Easter a boy on the ward came down with measles and we were quarantined.

NO VISITORS ALLOWED.

No matter how hard he tried, Uncle Harry could not find a way to sneak inside. He made up for it by coming every Sunday to the window at the end of the long room. The ward was on the ground floor of the hospital and my bed, this time, was at the very end. By making signs and signals and by shouting a little, Uncle Harry could talk to me through the window.

It was warm. On the Sundays that the window had been left open to air out the ward we could carry on a normal conversation in low tones with Uncle Harry ducking behind the lilac bush every time a nurse hove into sight.

Easter was late this year. The ward was very stuffy and a nurse coming on afternoon duty stepped over and flung the window wide. "A little fresh air doesn't hurt the measles any," she declared.

By now six or seven of us were covered with red spots. To be feverish and have a sore throat and rash, that was bad. But to be getting better and still quarantined, without visitors on a holiday, that was worse. Most of us were feeling very glum.

No sooner had the nurse gone out than we heard a whistle at the open window. It was Uncle Harry with an enormous basket of colored Easter eggs! Three or four dozen at least.

One by one, he handed them in and as quick as they were passed from bed to bed down the long ward, they were peeled and gobbled.

"Tell your friends to do something with their egg shells,

every speck of them,'' he admonished me before he left. ''I won't be your good old Uncle Harry if those nurses catch me.''

How to dispose of the shells, that was the question.

''Pass 'em down to me and I'll stuff 'em in the water pan behind the radiator,'' called Tony, a boy on the far end of the ward. ''They won't be turning the heat on until fall and by that time none of us will be here.''

When the dinner trays arrived, there was no sign of colored eggshell anywhere. Our appetites were poor but nobody chided us. Even the toughest nurse showed sympathy for kids getting over measles. When one came to take the trays away, she sniffed suddenly and looked around.

''It was chicken croquettes for dinner tonight, but I'm sure I smell egg.'' After inspecting a bedstand or two she departed with the mystery unsolved.

In a few days my rash was gone. Mom came to get me and I was on my way back to South Dakota, after six months in the hospital. In the middle of the night I awoke in the lower berth of the train and laughed out loud. I was remembering all those eggshells stuffed behind the radiator.

This time I could move a few steps with braces on, if I held onto the back of a chair for balance. I fell many times. I had to wear them, there was no way out. But most of the time I gave up bothering to shuffle those few inches and, with braces on, took to my wheelchair.

Inside the house, I found another way to get around and, at the same time, to strengthen muscles. Dad sawed a two-foot chunk off a log. He brought it inside and set it on the floor. Next he lifted me off the couch and showed me how I could, with the help of my one good arm, raise myself onto the log and roll around for short distances.

Summer was full of good times. Floyd and Jack tied me into the buggy and took me gopher-hunting with them. Practically everywhere they went, I went too. I went to the Fourth of July air show with them and, as I watched the stunt pilot do tricks, I vowed out loud, "Some day I'm going to fly. Just wait and see . . . some day I'm going to fly!"

When he heard that, Floyd laughed, but Jack believed me. Mom did too. "You've got a mind of your own, Don. And if you want to fly enough, no doubt you'll find a way to do it. Why even when you were a little tyke, half dying of polio and paralyzed from your neck down, you made a choice for youself. The nurse asked you what dessert you wanted—ice cream or jello, and you told her right out, "I'll take jelly."

Recalling the incident, she smiled.

These days Dad was involved in something mysteriously secret and exciting. It was called the Drake Estate. He went to lots of meetings about the Drake Estate and then he'd come home and tell the family all about it. We listened, wide-eyed.

We'd never heard anything like it before. It seemed almost too good to be true. In the not too distant future, my father was going to get a bundle of money, just from participating in the Drake Estate. He'd talked to other sensible farmers like himself and they agreed. They had gotten involved themselves because the deal was too good to turn down.

Dad told us people by the thousands were going to the meetings in different states, mostly the midwestern states like Iowa and the Dakotas and Kansas.

This was the story as he pieced it together for us. At the end of the sixteenth century, when Sir Francis Drake died on board ship in the West Indies, he had spent his pirates' booty on bigger and better ships. But a rumor circulated that Drake had left an enormous fortune. Some said it was as much as $22,500,000 in Peruvian gold, Oregon redwood forests, or Egyptian cotton fields. No one seemed certain which it was. But authorities were of one accord on the fact that the estate had been left unsettled through the years. Since Sir Francis Drake had been a British subject, of course settlement of his estate must be done in the British courts.

"What does that have to do with anybody in South Dakota?" Mom queried when she first heard about the Drake Estate. "How can we benefit from something going on in England?"

"Don't you see?" asked Dad, eyes ablaze with excitement. "Why lots and lots of people over here are descendants of Sir Francis Drake and can lay claim to some of his fortune." He paced up and down our small living room, then absentmindedly rolled himself a cigarette. This he stuck into a pocket to smoke later, outside. "Son of a bitch, *I've* got English blood in me, and Missus, you do too. You know you do! Why we might stand to gain thousands of dollars, if we scrape together a little money to contribute to this man Hartzell who's heading up the thing."

"I can tell you more as soon as I get back." With that he grabbed his hat, smashed it down on his head, and took off for another meeting, leaving Mom more than a little dismayed.

Despite current political efforts to deal with the farm crisis during the depression years, nobody had much money.

By suppertime when there was still no sign of Dad, my mother snorted, "That Kirk! Getting all excited about a fool thing like this!"

But before long, she became a firm believer in the Drake Estate, too. It turned out to be something to hold onto when the going got rough and a body thought there was little use in going on. The Drake Estate was like a marvelous dream that you sensed in your bones would come true some day.

In times like that, with no jobs to be had, and the land so eroded and worn out, and the drought and the dust storms on top of everything else, people needed a dream.

News about the Drake Estate passed from mouth to mouth. People talked about it in hushed tones. It was the gossip of church socials, picnics, bridge parties. Nothing could be printed in the newspapers about it. All meetings were secret. People heard by word of mouth when the next one was to be held. Whenever Dad said he was going in to town "to get the news," we knew he was referring to the latest on the Drake Estate. The settlement, which had to take place on the other side of the ocean, in England, had been delayed so many different times that nobody wanted to slow it down any further.

It was said there would be two groups of benefactors: those who were able to lay claim to the name of Drake somewhere in their family tree, and others who put up money to help a "rightful heir" who then promised to divvy up his wealth later on.

Dad had papers to prove the story was true. Somehow, some-where, he scrounged cash to take to each meeting so he, too, could be counted among the lucky benefactors when the great day arrived.

Often he came home from a meeting buoyant. "I'll wager it will be soon now, mark my words." At other times, he seemed disappointed. "Si Nelson claims a secret court is holding up the works, until the King can put a golden seal on the right papers." Or: "Oscar Proudhammar tells me a big group of people are trying to keep the money out of our country. No wonder the gol darn thing is going so slow!"

My second brace was getting too small and I was fighting against the prospect of returning to the hospital for a third visit when Oscar Merrill Hartzell was convicted of fraud. It was in the headlines of the newspaper. I pored over the story alone, not want-ing to look at my father and see his hurt. Hartzell was sent to Leavenworth, but Dad and many of the others refused to quit believing in the Drake Estate. Another man took over for Hartzell and, for a while at least, there were more secret meetings.

"I know it's true, this Drake Estate," Dad said firmly. "It's got to be. The whole idea makes sense. You'll see!"

I was firm about one thing myself, and it wasn't anything to do with the Drake Estate. "If I go back to the hospital," I told him darkly, "it's not going to be for any operation. Just for a new brace. That's all. And if nobody else tells the doctors, I will."

It was winter before I had to go. This time the doctors did not have it in mind to cut into me. But they soon decided to do something that hurt as much as that. Several doctors studied my twisted body. Then, after conferring with one another, they took me down to the hospital gym. They had decided to straighten my back by hanging me from a special frame for a period of time each day.

The frame had a padded chinrest with a metal piece around it through which my head could fit. When the nurse pulled the cord on the pulley and raised me up, the complete weight of my body was on my neck alone.

I heard a snapping sound. The pain was excruciating. Like knives going through me, a pain worse than I had ever felt before.

I gasped for breath. "I'm . . . I'm dying . . . oh . . . ooooooh, please let me down, please!"

That first day's treatment took but a few seconds and then I was back on the stretcher again, my entire small body screaming with pain. Each day after that, I was taken down to hang in the gym. It was only for a minute or two at first, then for longer and longer periods of time. At the end of three months, I could swing back and forth without a bit of pain and I hung there for twenty minutes at a time.

The treatment was considered a success. My deformed back had become much straighter and the doctor was pleased.

The hospital gym had other equipment, bars and a swimming pool, in addition to my hanging frame. I looked at the pool with longing every day when I went in for my treatment. How I wished I could swim! One day I asked about it. "Couldn't you let me get in the pool? Just once?"

"Don't be silly," scoffed the nurse. "You'd drown, you know that!"

Of all the doctors on the hospital staff, Dr. Williams who attended me was the only one who took Sister Kenney seriously. He pored over articles about her and told me about them.

"Perhaps the day will come when we use some of her methods here," he said. "She has some strange ideas about the value of water therapy for polio cases, Donald. Our president, you know, had polio a while back. But of course it hasn't left him with such bad effects. You can see by the newspaper photos how erect he stands. . . .''

Secretly, I wished he would go ahead and try something new on me. But I gave up any notion of getting into the pool.

Between hangings, I lay on the Older Boys Ward and stared out of the window, dreaming of what I would do when I grew up. The hospital was situated on a hill overlooking the river. A road ran along the edge of this river. From my bed I could see the cars go by. When the headlights flicked on at dusk, it was a pretty sight.

I thought of the things I wanted to do and be. A fireman or a cowboy . . . I put those ideas out of my head. Next best thing would be a pilot. I'd been reminded more than once, however, that piloting a plane would certainly take two hands and two legs.

Maybe I would be a lawyer. At home, Jack and I had invented a marvelous game. On long afternoons when snowdrifts outside the house prevented me from playing with the other boys, Jack often chose to miss a snowball fight and play this game with me. It was a game of law, a Perry Mason type of fantasy.

Since Jack was older than me, he almost always got to be the District Attorney. I was the Defense Attorney. After making up a theoretical case, we were off, arguing by the hour. If supper interrupted, we didn't mind. Afterward we took up the game where we'd left off, and argued until bedtime. Admittedly, Jack won most of the cases. He lied, sometimes, but I didn't care because the game was so much fun.

My mind flipped back to the present. Well, if for some reason I couldn't study law, how about being president? The grown-ups talked about Franklin Roosevelt all the time. He'd had polio and there he was, running the whole country!

Now that I was older, I was growing less patient with the

Victorian stance of the hospital. Everything was so tiresomely regimented. The tiniest infraction of the tiniest rule caused a furor every time.

One morning, as a nurse set my breakfast in front of me, I jerked a hand and over went my glass of milk. It happened quite by accident but that nurse thrust an angry face within an inch of my own and shook her finger at me.

"You did that on purpose . . . you spilled the milk!" she scolded.

For once I looked her in the eye. I did not recognize my own voice when it came out strong and clear. "Yes I did," I told her. "I spilled the milk. And what are you going to do about it?"

That was thinking for myself all right! Sort of like the time I'd decided about dessert in that other hospital so long ago. Or the time at the air show last summer when I announced to my brothers, "I'm going to fly some day."

I was beginning to have a little hair on my belly!

It came to me that a person's ability to decide had a lot to do with the way things turned out for him. Whenever I decided something for myself, it enhanced my sense of identity and put new power within reach.

Other experiences had an opposite effect. Especially one. While I was lying on a stretcher in the emergency room, waiting for a doctor to come, it happened. The nurse, a chubby girl who looked plain and uninteresting, was the only other person in the room. Without a word, she came and stood close to the stretcher. Keeping her back to me, she turned ever so slightly. Suddenly she reached underneath the sheet and fondled me!

Terrified, I didn't know what to think.

As soon as she heard the doctor's footsteps, she stopped. But in another day or two, she had herself transferred from day shift to night. Every night she came into the ward when the other boys were sleeping and stood by my bed and reached under the cover to touch me and excite me and terrify me.

Was I doing something wrong? Or the nurse? What made her do a thing like that? Who could I tell? Surely I'd be scolded for allowing it to happen. Remorse and guilt swept over me. My cheeks burned in the dark as I brooded over this strange occurence. No words passed between us at any time. It happened. That was all.

It was late in February and I was very homesick. Soon the chinook would be blowing in South Dakota. Maybe it was blowing now.

This time when I left the hospital I would never come back. No matter what anybody said or did to me, I knew I would never come again.

      " "PLEASE Donald. You've got a good brain. You'll never be able to get a real education stuck out on a farm like this. Mrs. Nelson told me about the Crippled Children's Home in Fargo . . . you'd live there and go to school. It would be a real fine opportunity. . . . "

Mom was coaxing again.

With Dad it was different. He merely said, "Look, son, why not go take a look at it. Fargo isn't the end of the world."

"If the school down the road is good enough for Floyd and Jack, it's good enough for me."

"Eight grades in one room," began Mom. "Sometimes you can only get there two or three times a week. And during the worst months, not at all."

Momentarily she gave up trying to change my mind for me. She found her hat and purse, took off her apron. "I'm going to club meeting. If I'm not back by five, you might start peeling potatoes."

Dad headed out to the barn. I knew I could holler if I needed him for anything.

I flicked on the radio on the kitchen table. During the middle of the day, you couldn't get anything but soap operas. Except music sometimes. I turned the dial, hoping I'd be lucky. A voice advertised Ivory Soap, 99-44/100 percent pure. And, on another dial, weepy old Stella Dallas.

I could hear Floyd out there helping Dad pitch hay. Jack had walked to town for a nickel ice cream cone. I longed to go lie down in the ditch Dad had dug for me at the side of the house. Earlier in the summer, he had filled it with water from our artesian well. Once the dirt settled to the bottom, it made a swimming hole for me. The rest of the family jokingly referred to it as my "hog waller." That was because I liked to stir the muddy bottom with my good hand. The oozy wet, muddy ditch felt mighty good in the heat.

Today nobody was around to lift me in.

I thought about Mom and how much time she had to spend lifting me in and out of my chair, off the floor, onto the couch, into bed. How time consuming it was for her to take care of me every time I sprained an arm or broke a leg when I tumbled. I was getting strong enough to do much for myself. But I could not get in and out of the privy alone, or take a bath, or navigate steps. When I fell out of my chair, I could not get up.

I felt unhappy with myself. The folks wanted to give me a chance for a good education and I refused it. They didn't want to get rid of me, I knew that. They were just wanting what was best for me.

Ugly memories of those three stays in the hospital whirled in my mind. I was certain I did not want to leave home again. Was that it? Or was I being an ungrateful brat? I felt unhappy with myself.

I took my Marine Band Hohner harmonica out of my shirt pocket and tried to cheer up with a tune. But first I polished it with my good hand on the leg of my pants. The harmonica was a treasure. Dad had gone down town and bought it one time when I was sick in bed. He could play himself, very well in fact, so he gave me a lesson and then let me figure out the rest.

Today I spit on it and shined it until it gleamed like a silver bullet in the palm of my hand. I played "Dixie" and "Jimmy Crack Corn," and "She'll Be Comin Round the Mountain." Then I played "Old Black Joe," a mournful melody. It made me feel bluer than ever.

After that I chose only rollicking tunes. I was working on "Oh Susannah" when Mom walked in from her meeting.

"Forgot the potatoes," I mumbled. "But I decided to have a look at that place in Fargo."

The only appointment Mom could get by letter with the chief doctor was for early morning, so we planned to spend the night in a hotel. When our train pulled into Fargo, she murmured in dismay, "I don't have any clock along. We'll need one to get to our appointment on time."

She clicked open her change purse to study its contents. Then she wheeled me into a department store where, to my surprise, she asked the clerk behind the jewelry counter to show her the cheapest wristwatch available. I was more amazed when she counted out two dollars and fifty cents, set the watch by the clock on the store wall, and handed it to me.

"You wear it, Don. When we're done with it, you may have it to keep."

"Golly! Gee whiz!" I couldn't believe my ears. A watch of my own . . . and it wasn't Christmas or a birthday or anything! If only the gang back home could see me now!

It had a black strap, my new watch did, and black hands, and small, clear numbers. It even had a minute hand. I kept looking at it while we ate supper.

"It took me exactly three minutes on the dot to eat my bologna sandwich," I told Mom. "But you took a whole ten minutes just to drink your cup of coffee."

84

"It was hot," she reminded me with a smile. "I had to let it cool."

At the hotel desk, my mother left a message for the bellboy to wake us. We went to bed early because we'd have to be up by seven. I couldn't sleep. I let my mother take my watch off to wash my face and hands. Then I put it right back on and took it to bed with me. All night long, I kept waking up and feeling the leather strap encircling my wrist. It was strangely comforting. In the dark, when I held it to my ear, I could hear it tick. Tick tick tick.

Minutes and hours were ticking by. Soon I would be in a strange new place. I'd probably have to stay there a very long time . . . days, months, perhaps years. Mom and Dad had explained that to me. I hated the thought.

"There's bound to be other boys like yourself, Donald," Mom had assured me. "Boys with crippled arms, boys in wheelchairs. Maybe some children who had the misfortune to be born with various deformities."

Sleepless, in a strange bed and a strange place, I thought about it. I was sure that was the one thing I didn't want . . . to be clubbed together with a lot of other kids in wheelchairs and braces. My own brace had come off for good a few months ago but not until it had rubbed huge boils under my arms. What I really wanted to do was to live at home, going to the little school with Floyd and Jack, making model planes and trucks out of scraps of cardboard and glue, playing the District Attorney game, and tearing around in the buggy shooting gophers like the other boys.

No chance of that. The grown-ups knew what was best, or thought they did. A few of my clothes were packed in the suitcase we'd brought and in a week or two, the rest could be mailed to me. A decision had been made.

When I saw the "institution" the next morning, I felt worse than ever. It looked foreboding.

"These places are always more cheerful when you get

inside," Mom told me. But a grim look came on her face when an attendant in a white coat showed us around. We were taken to a large main room. Shocked, we took in the unkempt children in drab hospital garb, children with listless limbs and vacant stares. We saw old men, drooling and jabbering in a crazy way.

"Pay no attention. A few of them are senile," explained our guide. "But nobody here is harmful."

We saw crutches and wheelchairs. Wheelchairs with pathetic creatures sitting in them, some grotesque in shape, others more normal, but all with sad, unsmiling eyes.

Mom was going to have to leave me here! Today! I swallowed hard. Pictures came to mind, kalaidoscopic fashion . . . pictures of Dad getting up early and going out to do the chores, pictures of Mom tossing corncobs into the range for kindling; Jack, a chunky kid, owllike in his thick glasses; Grandpa Merritt calling an auction; all of the little cardboard toys I'd glued so carefully, in a line upon the bedroom shelf; trucks with wheels that really turned too . . . I had figured them out by myself. I thought of the healthy gang of kids I played with . . . Mike and Soapy Wentworth, Jim Nelson, Leonard, Jake.

Oh no. This couldn't be true. But it was!

Our appointment with the doctor turned out to be brief. Mom asked a few questions. The doctor, guessing her first impression of the place, explained: "Most of these children are orphans. They have no relatives to care for them. The derelicts . . . well . . ." he dismissed the question with an embarrassed cough. "Where else could they go?" he said helplessly.

I felt cold all over. I looked at Mom. How soon would she leave me here and head home? Maybe I could persuade her to spend one more night in the hotel.

"Thank you for the appointment," I heard her tell the young doctor. Her voice was crisp. "After seeing your institution, I realize it is not the place for Donald. If you'll pardon me, we must hurry to catch our train."

I was going home! I wanted to sing and cry and shout all

at once. The only thing I managed to say on the way to the station was, "Oh Mom, it was terrible!"

"Yes," she agreed. "It was terrible." Tears sprang to her eyes. She wiped them away and laughed a little. "I guess you got what you wanted, anyway, Don. You're going home."

"The place wasn't fit for pigs," she told Dad the following day.

"Was it that bad?" Jack asked me, awed.

We were well out of earshot so I let him have the truth. "You're gol darn right it was. I don't want to talk about it or think about it. Let's get the buggy and go out for a little target practice."

The words *hospital* and *institution* were not mentioned again for many a day.

My wheelchair was falling apart. Long ago, the tires had worn off. Ever since, I'd been riding on the rims. That didn't bother me too much. I could go fast without tires on the thing. But other parts of the chair had been broken and mended many times too. I wasn't sure it could take any more mending. I showed it to Dad.

"Don, you do need a new chair. This old thing isn't good for much any more. Can you make it do till I pay a few bills? Another month or two?"

Mom came up with another idea. "Why don't you write to the newspaper? They might publish your letter. People reading it would get interested and give money."

She found clean paper for me from her kitchen drawer, and loaned me her fountain pen. "Make it neat, Don, so they'll be sure to print it. And why don't you address it to the Sioux City *Tribune*, in Iowa? That's a much bigger town than Woonsocket or Cuthbert. More people will see it there."

I labored over my letter for a good part of the afternoon. I wrote a rough draft through, with many crossings out, then copied it neatly in my best handwriting, without one misspelling. My old chair needed another welding job on the wheels, so it

was Jack who offered to walk in to town to the post office with
my letter that very afternoon.

The letter was published. A few weeks later, I had a brand-
new wheelchair. It was a beautiful, four-wheeled chair, two small
ones in front and two very big ones in back. It would not tip
like the old one. The tires were strong, the wooden seat and arms
sleek and shiny.

"Golly!" I exclaimed when I saw it. "Oh golly! I can really
go places now!"

Dad ran his finger across the satiny wood before lifting me
into the chair. "Softer than a schoolmarm's tit," he muttered, giving me a wink.

Mom glared at him but he paid no attention. "All set for
a ride, Don?" He farted loudly as we went out the door.

Roosevelt had been doing his best to wipe out the farm crisis.
Organizations were cropping up by the dozen, it seemed, to act
as spokesmen for groups of farmers. There was the Farmer Labor
Party, and the Farm Bloc, the American Farm Bureau Federation,
the Grange, and the Farmers' Union. Many more . . . I couldn't
keep track of the names but I liked to listen to Dad jaw back
and forth with other farmers when they met.

One night I heard one of them say Roosevelt had offered to
pay the farmers *not* to cultivate part of their land. It sounded crazy
and I said so.

"We're also going to get paid to rotate our crops and to try
a new kind of plowing . . . contour farming, it's called," said
Si Nelson. He spit a squirt of tobacco juice and hit the side of
the barn.

"New ways of farming make sense," I told him. "But how
can you get paid if you let your land sit for a whole year without
any kind of crop on it?"

Dad spoke up. "The land's worn out, Don. You can see signs
of that yourself. But farmers keep right on planting crops on it

anyway. They know the land won't produce the way it used to, but they have to keep on. It's been proved, though, if a farmer lets a field lie fallow for a time, his soil will improve. So Roosevelt is making it worth our while to do that. Like Si says, he's going to pay us not to plant some of our land.''

The newspaper told about the poorer families all over the country who were packing their belongings into old, broken down cars and moving farther west to California and Oregon.

"Will we have to do that?'' Jack asked at breakfast one morning. "Teacher says there's a nickname for it—Okies.''

"We're not Okies,'' Mom told him firmly. "We may be poor, but we're not Okies. Your father is a tenant farmer, not a sharecropper like those Okies. He's always paid rent for the land he farms.''

"We've moved around plenty,'' Floyd pointed out.

"It isn't the same,'' said Mom. "There's another difference. It's . . . well . . . it's cultural. We read good books. You don't hear your father or me use words like 'ain't' or 'goin.' It's hard to explain, but there *is* a difference,'' she ended lamely.

Dad had set great store by the Drake Estate. Now it looked as if nobody would be getting a share of money from it for a while at least. Not until Hartzell got out of jail and found a way to prove he was right. Dad stuck the slip of paper, which told about his own share in the venture, carefully in the top dresser drawer in the bedroom. It would keep.

Sometimes I saw him stop what he was doing and stare off to the horizon.

"I don't have time to wait,'' he muttered one day.

"For what?'' I asked.

Dad started. He hadn't realized I was outside in my wheelchair.

"For the land to restore itself. Even a powerful man like Roosevelt can't work fast enough to do that. It will take time as well as money and good planning. Years, in fact.''

For a minute we were both still, harkening to the silence. A clear voice bit into it suddenly. "Su . . . eeeeee. Su . . . eeeeeeee."

Dad laughed and I called, "Hi, Ollie."

The voice called back, "Hi, Don, that you?" And then "Su . . . eeeeee." It was the younger of the Nelson brothers, throwing scraps to his hogs. The Nelsons lived almost two miles from our farm, but voices carried across the open countryside. Ollie sounded as if he might be only two feet away, rather than two miles.

In a few minutes a woman's softer voice could be heard as she fed her chickens . . . "Here chick, chick, chick, here chick, chick, chick." Who was it? I wasn't quite sure.

Dad ground out the butt of his cigarette. His eyes burned and his face looked harsh, mean almost, seamed by weather and troubles. I knew he wasn't mean.

"I got to go talk to the Missus about something, Don," he said at last. "You want to stay here or come with me?"

When he found Mom, he told her it was time to make a change. They argued back and forth, and she wept. She hated to leave her friends. Dad stalked off without a word. He knew better than to mess around with Mom when she was working up one of her scenes. It wasn't long before she brightened and called him back.

"All right then, Kirk. Let's move to Parker. At least there we'll be within visiting distance of your folks."

I heard them in the bedroom, laughing and talking and making plans.

Parker was much larger than either Woonsocket or Cuthbert. It had several thousand people in it and it was the county seat. The courthouse sat on a steep hill with its front door toward Main Street.

"The guys that have money live near here," Dad told us as we hung out of the car windows to look. "You can lay a bet on it, anyone driving a cadillac is somebody in this town."

90

Two different railroads ran along each side of the town. Across one of them was east Parker, where the poorer folks lived.

"A town this size should have a decent grade school for Don," said Mom with satisfaction. "Being in town I hope he can go more regularly, not just two or three days a week. And of course Jack will be starting to high school with Floyd."

I had forgotten about that. Who would take me in and out to classes and to the toilet when I needed to pee? In the little schoolhouse it had always been Jack. Until now he'd been around whenever I needed help. What would I do?

Before Mom found an opportunity to go down to the grade school office to register me, three members of the school board came to visit us. They sat stiffly on our living-room couch, looking uncomfortable and a little sad. From the downstairs bedroom, I watched and listened.

One of them cleared his throat. "It has been brought to my attention that you folks have a son in a wheelchair. It is our duty to inform you he will be unable to attend school in Parker. The boys and girls his age . . . seventh and eighth graders . . . move from class to class throughout the building. The stairs are steep. Some classes are on the top floor and some are on the first. The . . . ah . . . the bathroom facility is in the basement of the building."

A shocked look passed between Mom and Dad. They'd counted on me being able to go to school. And so had I. I was dumbfounded. What a gyp! Some kids didn't like school but I loved to do sums and read. I was good at my studies, too.

"Perhaps we can think of a way to work things out," murmured Mom.

"Not in the present building," another school board member told her gently.

"It may be a different story when we get enough funds for a new school," ventured the third.

That was silly. I couldn't wait for a new school to be built any more than Dad could wait for the land to heal itself and produce good crops. Besides, how many kids in Parker were in wheelchairs? Probably none except for me. When they did collect funds, nobody would think of designing a new school to fit just one boy like me.

September came. It wasn't easy to watch Floyd and Jack purchase fresh, spanking clean notebooks and rulers. I watched them sharpen pencils with a jackknife out in the kitchen. I wanted to go with them. Oh how I wanted to go to school! But as long as we lived in Parker, there would be no school for me. The high school was as bad as the grade school. Lots of steps inside the building. Floyd and Jack had been down to inspect it.

What could I do to change the fact? Nothing. There was no way out but to accept it. Anyway, I could read books by the billion at home.

Not long after classes started, a teacher came to our door. She introduced herself: Miss Murty. She sat primly on the edge of her seat to explain to my mother and father she was willing to come by after school every night to help me keep up with my lessons.

"Will the school board pay you to do this?" worried Mom out loud.

"No, I'm sure they won't. No funds are available."

"But we don't have any extra money either. We've just moved here and my husband doesn't have a job yet."

"That won't matter to me. I want to come."

She had a plain face. Her mouse-colored hair was drawn back into a severe bun. She was an old maid with horn-rimmed glasses and bad breath but she flashed a smile at me and I loved her on the spot.

I had a teacher! And I would have school books and homework to do like my brothers. For seventh grade at least, I would be getting credit for the courses I took with Miss Murty. Roosevelt was doing his best to find jobs for people. Dad and Mom thought the world of Roosevelt. Why, he was almost like

God Almighty, Roosevelt was. One thing he'd done already and that was to dream up something called the WPA. Through the WPA, Dad got a job as superintendent of public grounds.

Different ethnic groups had settled in Parker. Mennonites, Germans, people of Polish and Swedish descent. We heard much name-calling and a constant war going on between Protestants and Catholics. Those of the younger generation had confused the matter by marrying into one another's families.

Parker had four creameries, each with its own truck, and, as well as the two railroads running along the edges of town, a busline came through it. This busline was owned by a character I wanted to get to know. The character was Judge Pezenik, the shrewdest lawyer for miles around. Pezenik was one of the rich guys who drove a Cadillac.

"That old geezer owns half of Parker," one of my new chums, Mike Crukshank told me. "He even owns the whole busline. You know how I found out? My Pop's a driver on the line. He tried to help old Pezenik up the steps one day and the Judge chewed his ears off. Mean? I'll say he's mean. Pop complained to the boss down at the station and the boss just laughed and said, 'Nothin I can do about it, Joe, he owns the whole darn line.' "

Judge Pezenik owned something besides Cadillacs and buslines. That was why I longed to meet him, no matter how ugly he was rumored to be. Tied onto the back of his sleek black Cadillac each time it went up and down Main Street I had seen a wheelchair.

"Sure he's in a wheelchair," said Mike when I asked if it was the Judge or someone else in his family that used it. "You mean you haven't seen the guy yet? He looks . . . sort of like an ape. Long arms that curl backward like this." He contorted his body to show me. "And an awful big hump on his back. He's weird looking. And that temper . . . you wouldn't believe it. He called my Pop a bastard!" Mike went away, shaking his head in disgust.

A man who couldn't walk driving a car, a Cadillac? I'd never heard of such a thing. It was, Mike had explained, a custom-built job with hand controls.

I was determined to get acquainted with the Judge.

My own new wheelchair was wonderful. It set me free. It moved so easily I didn't need anyone to push, most of the time. I could go to the ends of the town, propelling myself with my good hand. Six blocks, eight, sometimes ten. The autumn air smelled biting—fragrant, laden with sunlight. Until the winter winds howled in from the plains and snow fell, I would explore every nook and cranny of Parker. My fox terrier, Zip, went with me.

When winter did come, part of Dad's WPA job was to superintend the flooding of a field for an ice rink. After it had been flooded, he bundled up in muffler and cap and mittens and stayed there to make sure things went all right while people skated. Whenever it was clear enough for me to be outside, I took part in winter games.

"Hey, Don, come on out with us. We need you as end man in Crack the Whip." Jack's chapped nose looked like a radish sticking out above his muffler. He hunted for my cap and mittens and off we went. To spin around the ice in a wheelchair was almost as much fun as skating. Often I ended up breathless and laughing in a snowdrift.

Pretty soon I thought of a way to make money while the rest of the kids skated. It was simple. On clear days I could wheel myself downtown and buy up a big assortment of candy bars, three for a dime. I'd make a profit by selling them at a nickel each in the little warm-up shack at the rink.

"So you found yourself a job," said Dad when he heard my plan. "Donald, you're going to make out OK." His face looked impassive above the rim of his thermos cup but somehow I knew he was amused at me. And pleased.

The doctor in Parker had been a military man. Whenever anything was wrong with any of us, grippe or bronchitis, he strode into the house, ramrod straight, to check us over. A hard-boiled fellow, he didn't smile too often, but he was a good doctor. I liked him. Mom, though, was forever a jump ahead of him, reading about new methods and treatments that might do me some good.

"The state doctor over in the Sioux Valley Hospital has a fine reputation," she began one day. "He's the one who married my cousin, you know. I'll look into getting an appointment, Donald."

I was horrified. The word "hospital" had not been mentioned for many months. I'd decided I would never enter a hospital again.

Mom kept right on coaxing.

Huddled in the warm-up shack at the rink, I pleaded with Dad. He let me have a slurp of boiling hot coffee from his thermos before he plugged it with the cork and said slowly, "The Missus has a mind of her own, son. Why don't you go just to please her? Sioux Valley Hospital is only nineteen miles from here anyway."

In bitterness, I went, late in the spring.

The doctor studied me for a long time, trying to decide what to do. He called in other doctors to look at me and read my chart.

I whiled away the time getting acquainted. There was a ward of kids of all ages, but I didn't have to stay on the ward all day! Compared to the other hospital, this one was lax about regulations. I wasn't sick, so why should I stay in bed?

At home, my doting parents had continued to give me a great deal of assistance. But I'd grown strong enough at twelve to dress myself and to get on and off a toilet without help. The bathtub was another matter. I knew I might never master that alone. All in all, though, I was feeling pretty independent.

I discovered I could go any place in the entire hospital, up and down in the elevator, out on the hospital grounds, down to the gift shop to buy pop and candy . . . and no nurse yelled at me. I began to visit up and down the halls in various rooms. The long term patients were mostly people who were senile or old folks

95

with broken hips who, a nurse informed me, soon would become that way.

"Some day a medicine will be invented, something better than codeine, that a person like that can take to relieve the pain. For an old person in his eighties or nineties, a broken hip takes months to mend, and sometimes it doesn't ever heal. The pain is so nerve wracking that finally . . ."

"Finally?"

"They end up going crazy."

In my travels through the hospital I came across an elderly lady from Parker, my town. She had a broken hip. She was lonely, Mrs. Frazier was. She babbled without stopping for breath whenever I went in.

"Oh the pain! The pain! It's killing me, I tell you, why can't they do something about it; Donald, go tell the nurse to get me another dose of that medicine she gave me last night, you say your room is just down on the other hall . . . oh my God, what pain!"

"Not room, *ward*" I told her patiently. But she didn't hear.

Pale blue veins ran like rivers. Her cheekbones stuck out, dark stones beneath translucent skin. Set into their sunken sockets, her eyes looked wild. I didn't like to get too near her bed, lest she grasp me with her thin fingers. Maybe if that happened, she'd never let me go. Spread out upon the pillow like the frayed feathers of a hen my mother had just plucked for dinner, her thin white hair had a sour smell to it. She was incontinent so at times her bed smelled also.

Often her jabbering made sense but suddenly she would turn from raving about her pain to strange and frightening warnings about the doctors.

"It's their fault, boy, can't you see that? I must get out of this hospital and go home immediately. They don't want me to live, they're devils, they're deliberately trying to kill me, my son is in on the plot, call the police . . . there's a number in the inside pocket of my purse."

96

She raised herself slightly, fumbled in the drawer of the night stand, but weakened and fell back upon the pillows, gasping for breath.

I wheeled down the hall to the nurses' station.

"The old lady's getting crazier every day," the nurse on duty told me. "Pay her no mind, Donald. Go visit somebody else for a change."

I wheeled away, wondering. Who was right? Could they really be trying to bump her off, since there wasn't much hope for a broken hip at that age? The doctor who took care of me was so mean I wouldn't trust him beyond my little pinky.

He was planning some sort of further surgery for me. I knew that because he'd mentioned it in front of me. But I had news for him. He'd never catch me to put me under the ether cone.

I took the nurse's advice and went to another room. And another and another. I played three games of checkers with a man in Room 238, but for the rest of the afternoon, I couldn't get old Mrs. Frazier out of my mind. On my way back to the ward, I stopped to chat with a thirteen-year-old named Dot. Dot had been recovering from a broken foot. She was ambulatory now, with the help of a crutch.

We talked about Mrs. Frazier for a long time. The next day she accompanied me down the hall to the old lady's room.

"A lot of the time she seemed to make sense," Dot whispered when we pulled ourselves away at last. "But that stuff about the doctors killing her . . . are you going to call the police?"

"Maybe yes, maybe no. I haven't decided. Suppose the nurse is the one that's fibbing and the old lady is right?"

"She sure likes to have you come visit, Don."

"Yeah. Her doctor told me I cheered her up more'n anybody and to go in there anytime I want."

"Well then, are you going to call the cops?"

"I tell you I don't know."

I stayed away from Mrs. Frazier's room for a whole day, thinking about it and trying to make up my mind what to do.

That night I fell into an uneasy sleep, still thinking. I dreamed terrible dreams about knives and surgery and someone screaming. Again and again, somebody rent the air with screams.

I was wide awake but the screams continued to crack the night in two. Voices talked in the lighted hall, footsteps hurried.

"It's Mrs. Frazier, she's flipped out," said the nurse making night rounds. "Go back to sleep, Donald, nothing's wrong, it's just old Mrs. Frazier."

For days after that she screamed. The nurses shut her door and gave her sedatives, but still periodically she screamed. Sometimes a nurse brought me a message: "Mrs. Frazier would like to see you." I would roll my chair down for a visit but I couldn't bear to stay very long.

One morning when I stopped at her door, my mouth dropped open in surprise. The bed was empty. It had been scrubbed. I could smell the disinfectant in the air. And it had been made up with clean sheets and a fresh, snow-white pillowcase.

I asked the nurse about it. "What happened? Did she . . .?"

"She didn't die if that's what you mean," retorted the nurse. "They moved her to another building, thank God for that."

I heard the screaming anyway, muted, from the other building. Dot heard them too. Sometimes we saw the nurses pause in the middle of what they were doing and listen for a minute. As time went on, the screams got noticeably weaker. There came a day when we heard them no more.

The state doctor kept talking about the possibilities of surgery for me. But no grown-up was going to put a knife to me again. I'd make sure of that. Could I run away? The idea whirled through my head. I set it aside. How far could I get on wheels? And where could I go? Instead, I began to keep my eyes open for a scalpel. If only I discovered where the scalpels were kept, I could swipe one, when the time came, and threaten the doctor with it before he had a chance to cut into me.

If I had to, I would kill him.

One day the drawer in the emergency room where I was taken

for checkups slid open. Laid out in a row with the other instruments a doctor uses—tweezers and such—was a small scalpel!

The drawer had no lock on it, nor did the emergency room. I took a deep breath, relieved to know I could reach that scalpel if necessary.

Before any operation could be performed, the doctor must confer with my parents and they must sign a release slip. I sat in on the conference. I was thirteen. Dad no longer talked to me as to a small child. In front of the doctor, we talked man-to-man. My father asked my opinion about the proposed surgery.

"After all, since the surgery is to happen to Donald, it is reasonable to give the boy a choice."

What a choice! Would I prefer to remain in a wheelchair for the rest of my life, or undergo a spinal fusion that would enable me to stand upright and move about with the help of crutches?

"Would I be able to sit down?"

"Of course not!" The doctor thought the question stupid. "You'd never sit down again but you'd be able to move around. You'd be rigid, but mobile to some extent."

"I can move now," I pointed out. I was thinking of the wheelchair, my chariot, and the way it had become a part of me. What could it be like to always be standing up or lying down . . . no more Crack the Whip, no more riding in the car?

Dad understood. He turned to the doctor. "I don't see much good would come of being able to walk, especially with crutches, if you couldn't sit down. I have to admit, doctor, I agree with the boy."

"Well yes," began Mom. I didn't tune in to what she had to say after that. I sat there in my chair, astounded. "Yes" meant she was on my side. My parents were letting me make a momentous decision about a very big thing! My good hand clenched the arm of my wheelchair. I was shaking with joy and didn't want the doctor to notice.

He'd grown livid with rage. "You let a *child* decide something like this?" he stormed. He paced up and down the small office for a minute before standing in front of Mom and Dad. "If I had a son like yours I'd . . . I'd have him horsewhipped every day!"

Neither of my parents could think of an appropriate answer. Wordless, they rose and pushed my wheelchair back to the ward. They had not signed the release for surgery.

In the next days, the doctor studied my case history all over again. He examined me thoroughly a second time. "Perhaps they will change their mind. Meantime, you've gained weight. You must go on a diet. We'd have to thin you down before an operation at any rate."

I looked down at my arms and legs. I had grown chunky, yes, from months of Mom's homemade bread and biscuits and pie, mounds of potatoes dripping with gravy, fried chicken, pheasant, puddings, stacks of pancakes and syrup. Nobody could call me a frail child anymore.

"Hmmmm," muttered the doctor. He scribbled out a diet for the nurse to uphold. Thereafter, my tray from the kitchen bore half portions of everything and never any fattening dessert such as cake.

Wary, I thought he might go through with my surgery without persuading my folks to sign the slip. Maybe he would forge it. I had another way to fix him now, aside from the scalpel. Every chance I got, I sneaked down to the hospital shop and loaded up on candy bars.

I gained three pounds. The doctor was mystified.

Strange feelings stirred within me. At times I remembered the nurse at the hospital in Glasgow, Minnesota, and the way she had touched me. I was growing up and had some of the same longings unfulfilled. Girls were no longer just people, they were *girls* . . . female . . . different from male. I saw something new when I watched the younger nurses, rosy-cheeked and laughing . . . the way their breasts curved to fill their starched white uniforms.

"Softer than a schoolmarm's tit . . . ." the phrase was Dad's.

100

Then, too, I noticed the curve of a leg when one bent to smooth a wrinkle from her stocking. She caught me looking and blushed. Another time when one came to straighten my bedding, I stuck an ice cube down her back and roared amid ensuing shrieks.

I could joke back and forth with the nurses. I was quick on the repartee. They liked that. They enjoyed teasing back. When one of them chucked me under the chin, I grew warm all over.

Dot went home to Fargo. You could be very lonely in a hospital full of people. Mrs. Frazier was gone too, and I could find nobody interesting to talk to. Mom and Dad had bought me a little radio. I kept it on my bedstand and, by the hour, I listened to it. The talk people. Like Arthur Godfrey. He made me laugh, the way he spoofed his advertisers. He got away with it though. Soap operas. Music. That was best. Music. Benny Goodman, Harry James. Music lifted me out of the chair and carried me far away. Like books, only better.

Lying in bed, with the radio turned low, I pretended I had a trumpet. I propped it against my weak arm . . . I'd learned to use that arm as sort of a tool . . . and made the fingers of my good left hand work the stops. I dreamed of playing a real trumpet one day. It could happen.

Between programs like Amos and Andy and Jack Benny, I heard scraps of news. What Roosevelt was doing to end the Depression. And all about a rising new power in Germany, Adolf Hitler.

I grew homesick. I wanted to be home with Jack. I loved both brothers. But Floyd was older, interested in girls now, helping Dad with his work. Among the kids, Floyd was the big cheese. I admired him. It was Jack who had become my playmate and companion, Jack who helped me in and out of the places I could not go alone, Jack who went over my homework papers and wrestled and teased.

I was becoming more and more restless. I'd been every place in the hospital, there was no new corner to explore. One day I decided to follow a nurse through the underground tunnel to the dormitory where she lived.

"I'm coming with you all the way," I teased.

"No indeed you aren't! The housemother would have a fit."

"I'm coming anyway."

The elevator hit the basement and out she got. I followed.

"Donald Kirkendall, go back."

"I won't."

"You will."

"Who says? You can't stop me. Ha ha ha." I was really laughing now, and she was too. She couldn't help it. She started through the tunnel. It led between buildings, under the street to the dorm. I kept following.

"*Donald!* I tell you . . . go back!"

But there I was, in the basement of the nurses' dorm. I looked around, fascinated. Pink undies and slips and stockings hung drying on the clothesline. One girl in a terrycloth robe and curlers was doing her ironing. She let out a little scream when she saw me.

"*Donald Kirkendall*, who brought you over here?" It was not the housemother but the head nurse from my floor who stood gaping.

"Didn't you hear my question? *Who brought you over here?*"

"I brought myself."

"You couldn't have."

"Yes, I did."

A few days after that the doctor decided there was no way to help me if I refused to have surgery. The folks came to get me and I went home.

*seven*

---

AUTUMN, winter, spring, summer melded, ran together like colors on an artist's palette. When I had nothing else to do, I drew pictures. I was good at it. My left hand was strong. But sketching didn't take care of the energy, the movement locked inside of me. I wanted to run or jump. Other boys went out for track or played football. What would it be like to make a touchdown . . . to skim over the field with the rest of the team at your heels? What would it be like to fly? Not often, but every now and then, a plane flew overhead. When I heard one, I wheeled down the ramp Dad had built at the front of our house, to watch.

Like all South Dakota farm kids, the boys around Parker had one favorite pastime . . . shooting gophers. I watched them go, knowing there would never be a day when I could walk aimlessly down a country road picking off gophers whenever I pleased.

At any rate, I was a good shot. And that was something. If the gang was going by car instead of on foot, either Floyd or Jack would boost me in and take me along. Sometimes on a Sunday afternoon, Mom consented to drive while the rest of us leaned out the open windows of the car to aim at the critters. Gophers . . . they were a plague and we could bump off as many as we wanted to in an afternoon.

"Let's stop at Farnsworth's farm," Mom suggested after we'd been out for a while on a Sunday. "I'd like to pick up some eggs."

Dad was along with us. He and old Farnsworth stood in the shade of a cottonwood near the house, talking. Mom went in to get her eggs.

"You out shooting gophers? Bah!" The old man spat contemptuously in the dust. "There's one of those critters here in the barnyard. Just look at the hole he's dug! I haven't been able to get him yet. You know how they do, Kirk . . . come out and sit up on their hind end and look at you so saucy. Blamed if I can get him."

"Hey, there he is. Let me have a try," I whispered. "Floyd, Jack, Mike, shut up will you?"

I pointed across the yard.

"Are you crazy?" asked Dad. "That guy is well out of range."

"I can do it," I insisted. My rifle was a little twenty-two Savage that Uncle Harry had bought years ago, hardly bigger than a BB gun. I aimed and took fire.

Dad chuckled. "See? He headed right for that hole."

"If you'll go look," I told him calmly, "you'll find that gopher dead as a doornail."

Dad walked over and sure enough, there he was on the ground. "Well I'll be damned!" muttered Dad, picking him up by the tail.


Summer had ended. The other kids were getting ready to start school. My friend Mike would be entering high school this year.

Oh how I wished I could go too. All day long, the other boys would be busy with classes. And in the afternoon there would be sports and glee club and different activities.

I brooded over it. A left-out feeling engulfed me. I tried immersing myself in books. *Swiss Family Robinson, Sherlock Holmes, Tarzan,* the plays of Shakespeare, *Life* magazine, anything I could get hold of.

Consumed by loneliness, I explored the farthest corners of the town on wheels. I talked out loud to my terrier, Zip, but he couldn't talk back. One day I took off and rode a mile out of town to the dairy my cousin operated.

"Got any ice cream?"

"For Pete's sake, tell the rest of the family to get out of the car and come in."

"I didn't come by car. I wheeled out."

"You're spoofing, Don, you've got to be." My cousin was flabbergasted.

No wonder the wheels on my second chair wore out! Like the first wobbly chair, this one had seen hard use. It was spending a lot of time in Red's auto mechanic shop these days.

"Ask him to get it done by tomorrow if he can," I pleaded with Floyd one day when he was about to head for the shop. "Without that chair I can't go anyplace."

I fooled with the radio, trying to find music. With music I could soar.

I would need money to pay for getting the wheelchair mended. Dad couldn't afford that expense over and over again. I needed money, too, to buy books and other things I wanted. I thought of ways to earn some. I had plenty of time on my hands.

One day I might sell my inventions. Idly, I leafed through a batch of drawings and designs, thinking about it. My best invention was the plan I'd made for the two front fenders of a car. Fenders were hollow, weren't they? So why couldn't they have a cover that opened, converting them into storage space for packages and small suitcases? When I heard about a car designer who was trying that on the Dusenberg, I felt secretly pleased. I'd thought of the very same thing a whole year ahead of him! And my design looked every bit as good as his, better perhaps.

"You have to be twenty-one to get a patent," Dad pointed out. So I set aside the papers and turned my mind to other ways to earn money.

I overheard a shopkeeper talking to a customer. "Know anyone who could deliver my handbills for me? Last kid I had moved out of town."

Hastily, before the customer could say a word, I interrupted. "I can do it."

The shopkeeper eyed my wheelchair. "How about the houses with steps?"

"I'll stick the handbills on the bottom step."

"Wind would blow 'em away, son."

"Oh gee, Mr. Topper, I'll weight them with stones. I'd like the job."

"You're hired."

For two bits an afternoon, I delivered handbills a couple of times a week. I knew many of the important people in town and where they lived. And, as I wheeled around delivering the handbills, I thought of another job.

I discussed it out loud with Zip. I could be a door-to-door salesman, like Dad had been in the Woonsocket-Cuthbert area. Sort of a junior Watkins man. But I would be my own boss and choose my own products. Excited, I mulled the idea over in my head. I figured the capital I would need to get started, and what products I would buy first. I went home and wrote letters and made phone calls.

Soon I was in business. I sold perfumes, inexpensive jewelry, greeting cards, stationery, neckties, and boxes of candy. In addition, I took on a magazine route. It was an easy way for folks to do their shopping without going downtown. They didn't have to set foot outside their house. They liked to see me come. I made money, especially on the neckties.

A city commissioner hunted all over town for me before a meeting one day. He had spilled coffee on his tie at lunch. When he found me, he bought a new tie and put it on. "I've been looking for you, kid, boy have I been looking for you!"

It was Halloween. All the little children in town had a party and bobbed for apples down at the Grange. I overheard Floyd and some other high school boys whispering about a prank they wanted to play. Would they actually follow through? I wondered.

Late at night, the citizens of Parker, South Dakota, heard a great commotion. The light on the sheriff's car flashed. His siren shrieked wildly as he raced toward the main part of town.

Dad flung open the door of our house.

"Jee-rusalem! What in thunder is all that about?"

Except for petty thievery, crime was unheard of in Parker.

"It must be something to make him blow that siren," worried Mom. "Where are the boys? Don's here and I think Floyd and Jack came in a little while ago. I'd better have a look upstairs."

"Wait Mom. Listen, there it goes again." The siren wailed, closer this time. Desperately, I tried to think of ways to detain Mom. I knew Floyd was not upstairs.

Somebody rapped hard on our front door.

"Just checking, Sue."

It was my Uncle Floyd, the chief of police, with the sheriff at his heels.

"You know that big road grader that was parked on Courthouse Hill? Apparently a gang of boys gave it a shove. They pushed it clear down into the middle of Main Street."

"Can't have a bunch of ruffians doing something like that in our town," added the sheriff hotly. "We're out to find them."

"Is young Floyd home?" asked my uncle.

"Yes."

"*Are you certain?*"

"You can go upstairs and check for yourself," replied Mom shortly. She hated to be doubted like that.

Up they went. I shivered. I knew Floyd had been in on the prank. Hadn't I heard him planning it with his friends?

"By gum, you're right," apologized the sheriff a few minutes later.

Uncle Floyd chuckled. "He was asleep in bed, the covers pulled up to his nose, looking as innocent as an angel."

I could hardly wait to get Floyd alone the next morning. "How'd you get up there without any of us knowing a thing about it?"

"Shucks, I just tore around to the back of the house and shinnied onto the roof over the kitchen and in through my bedroom window." He looked sideways at me and added, "I bet Uncle Floyd was onto the joke. He looked like he'd bust out laughing any minute when he saw me in bed."

A few days later somebody squealed. Five boys, including Floyd, were escorted solemnly into the courthouse where the justice of the peace reprimanded them.

"I hope you won't try something foolish like that again," Mom commented when it was over.

In private, Floyd chuckled. "It was worth every minute in the courthouse," he bragged to Jack and me.

The year after that he was out of high school and off to Minnesota to work in a government camp. Never mind, Jack was still at home to keep me company. I had turned fifteen and felt more restless than ever. Until the snow fell I could continue with my route. That is, on the days my wheelchair wasn't down at the shop for minor repairs. I didn't look forward to winter. I wanted to get out and go places and do things. I longed for something exciting to happen.

One evening a neighbor, Jim Handy, stopped by for a visit.

"Hey, Don, look what I found when I was tearing down an old house! You can fix it up and use it if you want."

He held out the pieces of . . . a trumpet! Dazzled, I stared.

"For me?"

"Oh, shoot. If you can get it to stay together, maybe you can learn how to play it. Tell you what. If you get this horn together and learn to play, I'll let you be in my band."

Many a time I'd listened to his band. He knew how I enjoyed music. But a trumpet of my own . . . right now? I must be dreaming!

Time had dulled the brass pieces. They were badly dented and the tuning slide was off. Every valve was stuck, the bell was disconnected at the base. I could find a way to sodder it. One of the braces to hold the bell in place was also broken. Nothing missing though, not a piece.

For hours, I worked on my trumpet. Using a liquid sodder and miles of electrical tape, I finally got it together.

"Listen to this!" Delighted with success, I brought forth a dreadful squawk.

"You sound like a sick crow," commented Dad. "Better take a lesson or two from somebody, Don."

Jack thought for a minute. "Say, I bet Mr. Lakowski, the bandleader at the high school, would give you lessons. His room is on the ground floor. Why don't you go down and check it out?"

The high school was only sixteen blocks away.

"Sure," said Mr.Lakowski, "I'll be happy to have you as a student. Come Mondays at five o'clock."

He was a patient man. It wasn't long before I could play something that sounded remotely like Beethoven's Minuet in G . . . Da di DA di Da di DA . . . dum ti dum . . .

"It *is* Beethoven's Minuet in G!" exclaimed Mom after I had practised for a few weeks. "I had a notion it was, ever since you started working on it. Why, Donald, that sounds real good."

"The darned bell keeps falling off, no matter how much tape I use. Do you remember where I put that tube of liquid solder?"

The battered trumpet became part of me like my wheelchair was part of me. As winter wore on, I lived and breathed trumpet. When I wasn't playing it, I was listening to Harry James on my radio. Or the great Satchmo. Or Henry Bussy or Clyde McCoy and his Wah-wah trumpet. Years of pent-up energy found a release in music. In music I could go places. Oh man, I could go to the ends of the earth!

"No ad libbing, please," begged Mr. Lakowski. He peered over the top of his glasses. "Stick to the notes before you, Donald."

Still, rather than plodding along, I couldn't resist jazzing up many of the pieces he gave me.

The WPA had instigated a recreational center in town. I hung around the building until I spotted the piano teacher.

"I need to learn how to read music. I need to know about timing. And chords. Will you give me some lessons?"

I could use only one hand on the piano but she taught me the essentials of music. I drank in everything she had to say and went away thirsty for more.

All day long my radio poured out the current hits. I paid careful attention to the way the pros handled their instruments . . . Tommy Dorsey and his trombone, Benny Goodman on the clarinet, Duke Ellington on the piano, back again and again to Harry James. Note for note, I learned his theme song, "Ciri Biri Bin."

Whenever the snow let up, I laid aside my trumpet and went down to the skating rink to sell candy bars or play games with the rest of the gang. Dad wasn't well this winter. He'd caught a bad cold earlier in the season. It had settled in his chest. He sneezed and coughed. Sometimes he stayed home in bed and let Mom dose him with hot tea and cough syrup. Those times I realized he must feel awful sick. Never had I seen my father stay in bed all day.

When the chinook blew and things thawed out a bit, he was still coughing. His eyes watered. His face looked strangely gaunt and palid, but red spots burned in his cheeks.

"You have more fever," worried Mom. She made him go back to bed. The doctor stopped by to listen to his chest. He spoke gruffly to Dad to get him to listen. "It's bronchial pneumonia, Kirk. You'd better get to the hospital."

Dad gave in. During visiting hours at the hospital, he fumed about bills. How could they get paid? And where would the family find cash for groceries?

"Never you mind," Mom soothed him. "Pay attention to getting well. We'll manage somehow."

The snow had melted. The days dawned cold, but clear. I bundled up and wheeled through town selling my products. For a month, I turned every penny I earned over to Mom.

Dad arrived home. He seemed as weak and wobbly as a new-born calf but he was on the mend. He marveled at the way the family had carried on in his absence.

"Donald helped a great deal," explained Mom proudly. "I don't know how we could have done it without that boy. Jack had classes all day and then homework. It was Donald's wages that bought the food for our table, Kirk, did you know that?"

For a whole month, the family had depended upon me to see them through a crisis!

"Now that you're home, Dad, the first thing I'm going to do is take my wheelchair down to be welded."

The chair was a sorry sight, the wheels out of balance, some of the metal parts broken. Mom drove me to Red's shop and waited outside while I went in to see him.

"Tell you what, Don," said Red. "This chair is beyond repair. I'm afraid it's time to get yourself a new one."

"Oh Red! Fix it up the best you can. Dad's been sick. I don't have any cash for a new wheelchair. Even the cheap ones cost an awful lot of money."

His brow furrowed. "Tell you what," he suggested presently. "If you'll help design a chair, I believe I can build it for you. In my spare time."

Together we drew up plans and took measurements and dis-cussed possibilities. We argued about front wheels and back, and kinds of material to use. We wondered where we could order tires.

While we were working out our ideas, the barber came into the shop. Interested, he looked over Red's shoulder. His eyes took in my beat-up chair with its bare rims and he looked at the plans again, impressed.

"That's something," he said. "That's really something, designing your own wheelchair, and building it, too."

"Cost too much for Don to buy another," explained Red briefly.

Once or twice a week, I stopped by the garage to see how my chair was coming along. He had mended the old one enough so I could use it until the new chair was ready. I didn't like to prod him too much. He had other jobs to do, of course, on people's cars and farm machinery. But every time I looked around the shop I could see no sign of my chair. Had he begun yet?

I talked it over with Mom before going down for the umpteenth time. "Something's brewing, Don," she said smiling. "You'll have to be patient a while longer."

My bedroom looked out upon the street. Early the following morning, she hurried into my room and leaned over the bed to pull up the shade. "Donald, hurry up . . . look outside . . . look, Donald, look!"

A red pickup was coming down the street toward our house. In the back of it stood one of Parker's young businessmen, hanging on to a brand-new wheelchair.

"That isn't the one Red and I designed!" I exclaimed. "Wow . . . what a chair!"

Mom laughed. "It's the one Judge Pezenik and I designed. The businessmen in town took up a collection and Pezenik called me into his office to ask my advice about it. He had it custom-built for you. Donald, he sent all the way to Ohio for those tires and the chain that leads from them to the crank. The entire town was in on it. But I have a hunch the judge paid more than his share."

Dad was standing behind her, watching my face. He lifted me out of bed and sat me in the chair. "This is as good a chair as you can get," he observed. "A padded seat. And padded armrests. And, look, Don, the crank makes it so you don't have to have a hand on the wheel.''

I ran my fingers over the armrests. Then I reached for the crank and made the chair move. I laughed for joy. "This one has a personality all its own. I think I'll name it . . . Josephine.''

Up and down the streets of town I went, trying out my chair. It was wonderful. Pretty soon along came a Cadillac and who leans out but the old judge. "Quite a chair you've got, my boy. How does it run?''

"Swell. Just swell.''

"Give me a demonstration. That's good! Now let's see it turn . . . hmmmmm!'' He drove off with a satisfied look.

Late in the spring I decided I was doing well enough on the trumpet to see Jim Handy about being in his band.

"Remember, you said to come back to see you after I'd learned to play.''

An odd look crossed his face. "Aw, I was pulling your leg, didn't you know that, Don? I already got a trumpet player and I don't need two of them.''

I never let on how disappointed I felt. I wheeled back home. That evening I played my trumpet for a long long time. I got into the music and stayed there. I wished I could stay forever.

Some of my friends played saxophone. And Carl Wilcox, a high school sophomore, played guitar. Now that I was getting the hang of the trumpet, I could start a band of my own! I began to track down more kids who played instruments. I found another trumpet player, three who played saxophone, the guitar player, and a bass. I knew a piano player, a boy named Shorty Long. Shorty was fantastic on the piano, but he seemed so quiet and withdrawn. Would he join our band? I asked him. Oh boy, would he! He had never played jazz but he'd have a go at it.

Where would we practice? Nine people couldn't squeeze into a little bitty living room. Picturing what it would be like, we laughed. While we were looking for a place, Jim Handy dropped by. He wanted to have the old trumpet he'd given me a year ago.

Crestfallen, I handed it to him. He had found it and had a right to it. But what would I do for a trumpet? My earnings had been spent on clothing. Dad was sick again. But as soon as he heard about Jim taking the trumpet back, he got out of bed and went to work for a week to earn me a good, secondhand horn.

"There," he said, sticking it in my lap. "That's more like it. Now you can go ahead with your band. Doc Selser owns the armory, by the way. He might loan it to you for your practices."

"You fellows may use the armory," agreed Doc when we approached him. "On one condition . . . no liquor, no funny business, understand?"

We locked ourselves in there, two evenings a week, so that younger kids wouldn't pester us, wanting to listen. Everyone in my band considered practice as serious business. Often we worked at it until two o'clock in the morning. One night Doc stopped by to see how we were coming along. Surprised by the locked door, he got suspicious and kicked it in. He was more surprised to find all nine of us deep in our music, arguing about the best way to do a certain piece.

After Shorty got into jazz, I saw I didn't have to worry. He had rhythm and he could ad lib and that is what jazz is all about. I discovered Shorty Long could write music as fast or faster than he could write words.

Myself . . . I was improving on the trumpet. Some effects were difficult to get because of being able to use only one hand. I couldn't use a regular mute. Gradually, I learned how to let the valves halfway up, producing the same effect. It was a much harder way to mute notes, but I practiced and practiced it. My lip muscle was growing firm and hard. At the same time, I was training myself to listen to the entire band, but also to each individual in the band. It wasn't long before my ear could pick up a particular saxophone. I could say, "That was supposed to be a sharp, Joe. Let's try it again."

At night when I went home to bed after a practice, I was high on music. It would be a long time before I slept.

114

Soon we thought we were good enough to play at dances. On weekends there was always a dance going on some place . . . in the Grange Hall, at the Armory, or in an Elks Club in a neighboring town. We asked around and got ourselves our first invitation to play.

As bandmaster I had to get the whole thing organized. What would we do for uniforms? The professionals in the traveling bands that came around usually wore tuxedos. Of course we couldn't afford a tuxedo for everyone. I decided I'd wear a white suit, with a shirt open at the collar. The rest of the band wore blue jackets and bow ties.

"No tie for me," I muttered to Shorty. "When they were straightening my back at the hospital, my neck stretched to a size seventeen. When I get a tie on, I feel like I'm going to choke."

"That's OK," he said quietly. "You look real snappy in that white suit."

It pleased me to know he thought I was handsome. Many other people had said the same thing. At times I wondered if they were just buttering me up and yet every one of them sounded sincere.

For years polio had left me with a deformed, concave chest, but all this trumpet playing had served as a form of physical therapy! It had developed my chest and filled it out. From the trunk up, I looked as normal as anybody else. I wasn't overly heavy but because of my muscular chest and heavy neck I needed large-sized shirts.

I had found ways to partially conceal my short, flaccid legs. I bought slacks that were good-looking and slightly longer than my normal size, to add a few inches to my legs. Most of the time I wore sandals because the doctors, in cutting the leg tendons, had made it so my toes became flabby and gradually curled under a bit. By wearing long socks and pulling them through the toes of the sandals, I had discovered how to hide this particular deformity.

"You're a good-looking young man," Dad had told me

115

earlier the same evening. "Dark and kind of swarthy. Masculine looking. You could date any girl you wanted, if you'd give it a try."

Maybe I looked like that on the outside. But, aside from laughing, teasing, platonic friendships . . . and I had plenty of those . . . I felt terribly shy with girls. Who would ever want to make love to a guy like me?

Both Shorty and I were nervous about that first dance.

The sheriff had told us if we gave a certain percentage of our night's take to charity, we would need no license. Our first evening was a success. The following week brought another invitation, and, after that, another. Soon people were coming in droves to hear us play.

Every chance we got, we listened to other bands and picked up tips. We listened to Lawrence Welk and his Hotsie Totsie Boys, broadcasting from the top floor of a feed and seed store in Yankton. We heard Happy Jack O'Malley, and the Rosebud Kids.

We got acquainted with members of the various traveling bands that came through town for a one night stand. Two different bands gave us the orchestration to sets of music they were no longer planning to use. We were thrilled.

"I say, Don, do you realize what we have here?" Shorty's eyes lit up. "These orchestrations would've cost us a pretty penny if we had had to buy the sets."

I felt good about them too. But my mind was on something else.

"I got a melody in mind for a theme song, Shorty. You want to write it down for me?"

The two of us had composed several of the pieces we'd played at dances. But this melody and words kept running through my head. Shorty hadn't heard it yet. He got a pencil and paper and lined it off into bars. Then he listened while I hummed the notes and told him the words I had in mind:

116

Yellow roses in your bouquet . . .
　You go passing by . . .
Yellow roses in your bouquet . . .
　O won't you tell me why?
Why do I think of you
　all night long and all day through?
Why do I sit and cry just because of you?

I was thinking of no particular girl, no particular yellow roses. At seventeen, I dreamed about falling in love. At the grange halls where we'd played, I'd seen boys steal a smootch or two whenever the lights got dim. I had watched the girls giggle and swish their skirts and flirt.

Would I dare ask a girl to go on a date? Most girls liked to dance and of course I couldn't do that. I felt crushed by the notion of a rebuff, so, for the time being, I did not bother to ask.

Surely some day I would find a very special girl, a girl I'd think of all night long and all day through. Meantime, I buried my longing in music.

We developed a good reputation. People came from miles away just to hear us. One day the manager of a talented young musician came to see me.

"Don, I got the most wonderful accordian player. He'd be great for your band. Can you drive over to Sioux Falls with me to hear him next Friday night?"

Twice I put the man off. At last he arrived at one of our Saturday night dances with his protégé in tow. During the intermission we had a one man show in a car in the parking lot.

"I have to admit, he's the best accordian player I've heard in a long time. But I can't use him right now."

The manager looked disappointed and so did the accordian player. "Jot down my name. Some day you might need a guy like me."

I took his advice and wrote it on a scrap of paper . . . Myron Floren.

It was the summer of 1939. A job at one of the local creameries opened up. Dad took it. It would be his task to test the rich milk the farmers brought to town and to pay them according to the cream content.

"At this salary, I couldn't turn it down," he told the family. He was going to earn sixty-five dollars a month.

In September, Hitler marched into Poland. After that, in quick succession, he took Norway, Denmark, and the Netherlands. We listened to Lowell Thomas on the news each night and talked about it some. But that was happening in Europe on the other side of the ocean.

"Jerusalem!" muttered Dad. "What kind of a man is he . . . this Hitler?" Abruptly, he switched off the radio.

"We don't have to worry about anything as long as Roosevelt is in office," Mom cheered him. She handed him a letter from Floyd. "This came today, Kirk. Floyd's got a girl in Minneapolis." She sighed absently. I knew she must be thinking of the way we were growing up so quickly.

It made things different, growing up. Jack was getting ready to graduate. He thought he'd like to try living in Minnesota too, for a while. My guitar player was in Jack's class. By fall he'd be off to college. And my drummer had taken a new job some place, so the band was falling apart.

When we began to disburse, I decided it was time to form a new band. At least Shorty would be around for another year. He promised to stay on as pianist. This time I gathered together enough musicians for a six piece band. We wore sports jackets instead of uniforms and we practiced in each other's homes, choosing the ones with only a step or two so that I could be hoisted in and out easily in my chair.

The members of this second band called themselves The Blue

Notes. We ad libbed more. All of us agreed, we sounded like pros. Before dances we'd stop at a café for coffee. Sometimes I felt a twinge of embarrassment when people watched me being carried in and out of the car or up a step. But I was learning to choose priorities. I didn't mind being packed around like that when I was leader of the band. I felt ten feet tall when I heard a pretty little sixteen-year-old say to her friend: "See that one with the trumpet? He's the band leader!"

She was talking about *me*.

Music was helping me to discover who I was. Alone for long hours during the day, I lapsed into a blue mood, wondering. But give me a Saturday night of trumpet playing and I knew . . . I was a bandleader . . . I was somebody. "Yellow roses, yellow roses . . . in your bouquet . . ." One of these days I'd find myself a girl.

One day a car salesman stopped me and said, "I've got just the ticket for you. A car with no clutch. It's hydromatic. You got to see it to believe it."

I was skeptical but went along. He wasn't fooling. It was automatic. I laughed out loud, excitedly. "I'll drive a car like this some day, it's great, that's what it is, great. There'll be a day when I can buy one for myself."

On December 7, 1941, the Japanese bombed Pearl Harbor. Stunned, we listened to the president's announcement on the radio. He had asked Congress to declare war.

My father shook his head sadly. "I suppose boys like Floyd'll have to go. If they don't enlist they'll be drafted soon enough. And things'll begin tightening up here in the states, mark my words."

His prediction came true. In the middle of April he came home from the creamery and said, "Well Missus, how would you like to go to Oregon?"

Mom's hand trembled when she put down her coffee cup. "Oregon? Do you mean it, Kirk?"

119

"Dang rights I mean it. Three of Parker's creameries are closing down. Including mine. There's shipyards in Oregon and plenty of jobs to be had. I've done a lot of other things in my day. I guess I can build victory ships as good as anyone else."

*eight*

---

" "W E have a week or so to get ready," said Dad the next morning. "We can only pack what'll fit into those two big suitcases in the hall closet. Come Saturday, we'll move the rest of the stuff into the front yard and have a sale."

"Thank goodness I've got time to write to Jack and Floyd and let them know what we're up to." Distracted, Mom wiped her hands on the end of her dress instead of her apron. "A week'll give them a chance to write back before we go."

Our house bulged at the seams . . . china dishes, sheets, pillowcases, towels, blankets, tables, chairs, rugs, knickknacks, pictures, mirrors, books . . . the accumulation of several years. All to sort out in one short week.

Long after I'd gone to bed each night, I could hear Mom's heavy tread as she moved about the house, folding clothing, packing and repacking the two suitcases, discarding letters and other treasures. It was hard to decide what to take and what to leave behind. She would have to sell her potted plants. I knew how much they meant to her.

Later the voices in the bedroom next to mine would start murmuring like running water, sometimes rising in an argument or laugh.

"I just hope you find wages as good as those at the creamery," I heard Mom say. "You'll have to go far to beat sixty-five dollars a month. How long will it take to drive to Oregon in the old Chevvy, Kirk?"

Turning over in bed, Dad muttered something but I couldn't make out his answer.

I thought about the Chevvy. It was nine years old but it would make it across the mountains. Dad had taken it to the garage for a tune up. He'd paid seven dollars for new tires.

Each one of us was busy, saying goodbye to relatives and friends, deciding what to give away, what to keep, what to sell on Saturday.

That day, when every bit of furniture and bedding, every dish, vase, and book had been sold, Dad smiled. He shoved his hat back off his forehead and sat down on the floor to count his money. Eighty-seven dollars!

"That gives us some to travel on, Missus."

Mom cast a tired glance at him and managed a smile. "Guess we can go over to your brother's for the night then, if there's nothing more to do here."

The house was an empty shell. I didn't want to wheel back up the ramp to have a last look. All the life had gone out of it anyway. I was feeling bad enough about Zip, my terrier, as it was. We'd heard dire reports of the terrible things that might happen when we crossed the border into Oregon.

The state police were rumored to be brutal. Somebody said they would kill any dog coming into the state. And so I'd parted with Zip, rather than have him hurt. Yesterday I'd scratched him in his favorite spot on the chest before I let some friends take

122

him away to a new home. He'd gone off, wagging his tail, not knowing he would never see me again.

It was a mixture of good and bad, this move. My chest ached with a tangle of feelings. It was bad about Zip, and about Dad losing his job at the creamery. But going to Oregon was exciting, new . . . except for trips to the hospital in Glasgow and that one dismal overnight stay in Fargo, North Dakota, I'd never gone out of the state. I had read about the northwestern part of the country in books loaned to me by Miss Murty. There would be an ocean somewhere near Portland. And trees. What would it be like to live in a real city? I would have opportunities to hear good jazz. Music, that's what a city would have. All kinds of music.

I had packed my horn.

One day left before our departure. And the best surprise happened. Jack suddenly appeared on the scene! He hugged Mom and Dad and whacked me on the shoulder.

"Floyd couldn't make it. He's going to get married before he goes in the army. But I'm going with you to Oregon. You didn't think you'd leave me behind, did you?"

When things had quieted down a bit, he confessed to Dad, "Really I was concerned about you making it across the mountains in the old Chev. Probably won't hurt to have an extra man along to help with the driving."

He helped Dad tie the two suitcases on the front fender with rope. Josephine, my wheelchair, had already been lashed to the back of the car. Early the next morning, my aunt cooked our breakfast and we took off on the dusty road out of Parker, heading west.

Every nook and cranny inside the car had been stuffed with small belongings that had not been squeezed into either suitcase. For the time being, Dad was jobless, we were on the road traveling. Nobody knew what was in store. We had not been driven off our land, though. We had made a choice.

Four days we journeyed, across the northern part of Wyoming, a corner of Montana, through Idaho and into Washington. At night we stopped over at motels, making certain to find cheap ones so our money would last, and also motels with a low step to accommodate my wheelchair. Sometimes my father drove. Sometimes Jack took over at the wheel while Dad snoozed in the front seat beside him.

We crossed the Rockies. South Dakota was far behind. By the third day, we'd run out of talk and sat with our hands in our laps, subdued, wondering what life would be like in Oregon. We were tired. Very tired.

"At least one good thing," commented Jack. "The only trouble we've had with this old car is a burned out generator. We're mighty lucky."

He was riding in the back seat with me for a change, and Mom was sitting along side Dad, talking to beat the band to keep him awake.

It was growing dark. We were making our way over a steep hill in Idaho. When we hit the next town we'd look for a motel. In the morning we'd head across the state of Washington and, by nightfall, down into Oregon.

There was no town in sight when suddenly the engine sputtered.

"Son of a bitch," muttered Dad under his breath. He rolled to a stop. Quickly, he got out and flung up the hood. A cloud of steam billowed into the dusk.

Dad came around to the side to talk to Jack. "She's out of water."

"That isn't so bad," replied Jack, relieved. "I'll get out and look for a creek."

Mom got out too. She walked around, stretching her cramped legs. Soon she climbed into the back seat with me.

"We'd better let Jack and your father take the front, in case we run up against more trouble along the way."

The two of them came back to the car with a coffee can full of water, which they poured into the engine.

124

"I'll drive a ways," offered Jack. By now it had grown very dark. Thinking Mom was still occupying the front seat, Dad flung open the back door of the car and crawled in right on top of her. She squealed like a pig getting butchered.

"I say there, you folks having trouble?"

The strange voice boomed out of the darkness. Headlights glared. A face leaned through the open window of the Chevvy . . . the face of a state patrolman!

We fumbled for words.

"Troubled? Us? No indeed!" Dad did his best to sound casual.

"Then if everything is OK, I'll be on my way. Saw the Dakota license and thought you might be stranded and need some help."

"Why for goodness sakes, he was perfectly all right!" murmured Mom in an astonished voice when we were alone once more. "He didn't act like a brute. He wanted to help us!"

Just the same, for a minute or two, we sat there shivering before Dad pulled himself together and started up the motor.


Rain. First a drizzle, then a downpour. We opened every window of the car and stuck out our hands to feel the wetness and to inhale the sweet damp air.

Mom sighed. "It makes the trees so green. So green!"

The leaves were already on the trees in Oregon, glistening with drops of rain against the somber April sky. Pale green leaves, and the darker evergreens.

We crossed the interstate bridge from Vancouver to Portland. Dad honked the horn and Jack yelled, "We're here! Wow! Look at the cars!"

We had turned onto Lombard Avenue. Automobiles inched along, bumper to bumper. Carefully, Dad maneuvered the old Chevvy into line. Someone honked angrily behind us.

"This is what is known as a traffic jam." Dad looked down

at his watch. "Five o'clock. People must be on their way home from work."

Mom pointed. "I see a motel."

But Jack's eye caught the sign: "No Vacancy." Slowly we moved on. Four more motels. All filled.

"It's wartime, ma'am, a lot of folks are traveling, you know." The last motel manager sounded apologetic. "You gotta start looking by three in the afternoon."

"Well," said Mom thoughtfully, "I have Ruth Mayberry's address in my purse. I haven't seen her since I left Iowa. Except for that one time she and Bud came through Woonsocket years ago."

"She might be able to steer us to a motel or rooming house," suggested Dad. He parked at a gas station and went in to ask for a city map while Mom hunted for the Mayberrys' address.

The lights had come on. Garishly, the colors reflected in the wet pavement, winked red, green, yellow. Sailors went in and out of taverns, some with girl friends brightly scarved against the rain. A man and wife came out of a grocery store with arms full of packages. A cop walked by and a newspaper boy, whistling, a fat lady with her arms full of packages holding a pink umbrella over her head, two little girls, an old man leaning on a cane.

Riding down the main street of Parker, we had known every person we saw by name. Here we were strangers. It was a queer and lonely feeling.

"Here we are . . . Chatauqua Boulevard," I sang out when I saw the street sign. Dad turned the corner and the four of us began looking for the right house number.

Mom was getting fidgety. "It's so late. And I haven't seen Ruth for nearly ten years. What would they think if we descended on them right at dinner time?"

"All right," Dad agreed, too weary to argue. "We can come back and pay a call on them in the morning."

"Where are we going now?" I asked. "I'm getting hungry."

"I could use a couple of hamburgers myself," admitted Jack. "Dad, why don't you drive back across the bridge to Vancouver. Some of those motels we saw out on the highway might have a vacancy."

Every one of them was full. But one manager said, "I've got a new cabin out back. It isn't finished yet. No heat. But it'll be a roof over your heads. I'll let you have it for half price."

Gratefully we paid him. Jack ran out for hamburgers. A little later, Dad and Mom and I squeezed onto the one double bed. Jack rolled up in a blanket on the floor beside us. We talked back and forth in low voices.

"All of those cars . . ." said Jack. "Never saw so many in my life. And with gas rationed like it is, too!"

"Did you see how green things look? One thing's sure. We won't have to worry about dust storms around here." Mom laughed nervously in the dark.

We lay awake talking for a long time, too excited to sleep. Excited and, I think, a little frightened.


"Why Sue Kirkendall!" cried Ruth when we stopped by the house on Chatauqua in the morning. "For land sakes!"

Bud was busy shaking hands all around and helping Dad and Jack lift me into the house.

"Why didn't you folks ring our doorbell last night? We'll be happy to put you up until you find a house to rent. I don't want to hear another word about it."

Ruth had the same friendly, talkative manner as Mom. All the time she talked, she was hustling around the kitchen, pouring coffee, setting out plates of donuts, deciding how she and Bud could double up to make room.

"You and Kirk can take our room; we'll use the roll-away; Don here, there's a single bed in Bud's study for him, and that leaves the couch for Jack. . . ."

Out in the living room, Dad and Bud and Jack were discussing jobs. I took in both conversations at once, but pricked up my ears when I heard Bud Mayberry say, "Three and four hundred dollars."

Presently Dad came and stood in the kitchen doorway. When he could get a word in, he said, "Missus, you didn't have to do all that worrying over the salaries being as good as what I earned at the creamery. Bud tells me the shipyards start their employees at three hundred dollars a month. Some earn much more than that."

Mom stared at him, speechless.

That very afternoon my father went out with Bud Mayberry. He came back exultant. He had a job.

"As soon as possible, I'll get on at the shipyard. Meantime, I'm starting at the chain factory under the St. John's bridge. They manufacture chains for victory ships."

"My stars," gasped Mom. "Do they take women?"

"At the shipyards? You bet they do. They'll take anyone they can get. They're so short-handed with men going off to war!"

A light glinted in Mom's eye.

I was doing some fast thinking myself. If they were that short of manpower, perhaps I could get on too. I could play a trumpet, draw, write letters with my left hand. I was eighteen. Why not?

In a month we were settled in our new house, one that Jack had found for us. Dad was already working at the shipyards now, and Mom too. She had traded her apron for overalls. But she didn't have to wear a hard hat like Dad. She was not involved in welding. She was a tacker. For eight hours a shift, she tacked two small pieces together so someone else could come along and weld them. She startled the whole family by taking up smoking. It was something to do on her fifteen-minute breaks, she told us.

My Bible quoting, Victorian mother with a cigarette in her hand?

But then, a war does strange things to people.

Jack was not around. He had gotten us settled, helped to build a new ramp for my wheelchair, and all this time he was busy memorizing the eye chart so he could get into the Navy. It worked. He had fooled them; he was in boot camp.

I was experiencing a loneliness worse than any I'd known before. Nobody my age around, and now to lose a fellow as close as Jack!

I had received a draft board notice too. We both chuckled over the sarcastic letter I wrote to the board before Jack took off.

"In answer to your letter of April 25th, I am not a conscientious objector. If at any time you can find a place in the army for a wheelchair with armor plate (you could possibly make a tank out of it) I am willing to leave at your convenience."

We laughed, but that letter went into the mail tinged with the bitterness I felt at being left out of the war. Never mind, I would apply for a job at the shipyards. There must be some kind of job I could do there.

"We have no doubt of your sincerity and capability," the man in the employment office told me. "But it would be impossible for us to insure a person in a wheelchair."

He looked at me with pity in his eyes. The pity did it. It brought to mind those early "poor Donnie" years . . . Preacher Hagglethorpe's sepulchral voice, the clucking of my mother's coffee klatch friends. Angrily, I wheeled out the door to the elevator where Dad was waiting.

"They wouldn't take me!" I told him why.

"Son of a bitch." He didn't try to baby me or ease my hurt. "Look Don, I'll drive you home and then I have to get to work. My shift starts at three."

Later, he said, "Portland's so much bigger than Parker. I'm sure you can find some kind of job if you try."

No offer to pull strings or to do some of the looking for me. I was a young man now and Dad respected me. Not once had he said, "Don, you need to be on your own," or "The Missus and I have supported you all these years . . . it's time to begin taking care of yourself for a change. . . ."

129

I knew he was waiting for me to make my own decision. He was not about to do it for me.

I had never seen anything like Portland. I was a dirt farmer's kid with cow pie up to my ears. I thought I'd been around some as a Saturday night band leader, but I soon discovered I had lots yet to learn.

I was an alien in a new land. The sights and sounds and smells of Portland were difficult to assimilate. Up and down the streets of the St. John's area I rolled, finding driveways when I needed to cross since I could not manage the curbs without help.

Both Mom and Dad were on swing shift, so the days were lonely and I slept. By four in the afternoon I was out gawking. People everywhere . . . the city was overloaded with an influx of people. From Oklahoma, Wyoming, the Dakotas, from as far away as Texas they came, looking for jobs in the shipyards. Gas rationing didn't matter, there were car pools. Cars were bumper to bumper when factories and shipyards let out. I'd never seen electric buses before, but I saw dozens of them now, with bodies squashed inside and more waiting in line on the street corners. I saw soldiers, sailors, marines going in and out of taverns and grocery stores, girls with tight, skimpy skirts and sweaters that revealed the full shape of their bosoms.

The streets were lined with trees. It was May and many of them were in bloom, ladening the air with a sweet scent. Dogwood, oriental crab, flowering plum, hawthorne. I learned their names. I drank in a mixture of new smells, besides the flowering trees and gardens . . . city smells of asphalt in the rain, gasoline, soot, and the heady, sweaty, sour smell of people.

Housing developments went up almost overnight, jerry-built, not meant to last more than a few years. Trailer courts did a thriving business. Newcomers to the city were willing to live any place they could find. I saw at least one trailer court where people lived in makeshift homes slapped together from pieces of corrugated tin, car bodies, anything.

The taverns held a mystery of their own. Whenever I found

130

an opportunity, I peeked inside their swinging doors. And the restaurants, clubs some were called. I had my favorites, like the Blue Lion, where I stopped for coffee and an eighty-five cent corned-beef dinner. The Blue Lion reeked with a pungent odor I soon identified as bootlegged whiskey. Fatty Johnson, the owner, admitted outright . . . he didn't have a liquor license. Nor did most of the other clubs like his. Why did I think he hired those two cops out front, anyway?

I conned the guy in the liquor store on the corner into thinking I was twenty-one, and got myself a license so I could sample some of Fatty's bootleg. You can't stagger very well in a wheelchair, but I got high and felt on top of the world. I made friends with everybody in the Blue Lion and boasted about the band I'd led back in South Dakota. I was no longer alone.

Almost every night after that, I made the rounds—the Blue Lion, The Purple Cow, Sparky Doolittle's, the Sunshine Tavern. Some of them weren't in the St. John's area but I'd park my wheelchair in a corner and take off in someone's car for a night of music and joking and fun.

I was learning the wartime songs—"Rosie the Riveter," "Harbor Lights," "White Cliffs of Dover"—when I had time, I'd practice them on my horn.

I met all kinds of people at the Blue Lion, especially after I'd played my trumpet there a time or two. Things didn't get started until around eleven o'clock at night when Fatty rolled out the gambling tables. Take your pick . . . black jack, straight poker, dice. He had one pool table, too. Mixed in with the sound of clicking dice, voices, laughter, was the music of whatever jazz band happened to be playing that night. In between the numbers played by the band, you could put a nickel in the jukebox. Delicious smells wafted from the kitchen . . . fried chicken, cabbage, meatloaf and gravy, laced with garlic and that pervading, strong odor of bootleg.

It wasn't long before I got acquainted with the Duchess, an old gal who was half oiled most of the time. The Duchess was

131

a regular barfly. She lived up to her nickname all right, she wore glasses and a tight girdle, and played good honky tonk piano. On the nights I played trumpet, I found it hard to calm her into supper music. Up close, I saw her the way she really was, a female past her prime, a wearer of old hats purchased at the Goodwill store, hands and arms loaded down with dimestore jewelry, stinking of cheap perfume. She overdid everything, especially perfume. There were times she came in smelling like an undertaker. Once I watched with my own eyes while she uncorked a new bottle of cologne from Woolworth's and poured it over her hands and face, laughing.

She had her dignity, the Duchess did. She wasn't flaunting sex like some women do. She didn't have any left to flaunt. I guess she knew that.

Among my buddies were a couple of merchant seamen. One, Mel, would tell wild tales after he got looped . . . tales of supply ships getting torpedoed right and left. A chill crawled up and down my back, farm kid that I was, as I heard the dangers a merchant marine must face during a war.

One night another seaman, Jake, had a fight with a sailor. Suddenly—*pow*—the guy's head hit the floor, scaring the hell out of all of us who were watching.

"He isn't breathing!" whispered an awed onlooker.

"Oh my God! He's dead!" moaned Jake, hiding his head in his hands. "I sure didn't mean to do that. What'll we do with the bloody bastard?"

Luckily the cops usually out front were no where in sight. Nor, at the moment, was Fatty Johnson.

"Tom and I can help you drag him out back," piped a voice from the crowd. "Why don't we take him around to the alley? Does anyone know his name?"

The sailor was nameless. And now he was dead. Weird thoughts ran through my mind . . . how would his family ever discover what became of him? They'd probably think he was missing in action. What if he didn't have a family? Would it matter?

"Guess what!" mumbled Jake coming in from the alley after a few minutes. "We were out there, all of us, trying to decide how to hide him in the bushes without too much commotion and what happens? The corpse shakes his head and wakes up! The guy ain't dead after all. Joke's on me I guess."

His laugh sounded hollow. It was a while before I noticed the color coming back into his pallid cheeks.

One fellow I didn't care for much, a huge, barrel-chested brute about six foot three. We called him Tex. He swaggered in and out of bars wearing a white ten gallon hat and a leopard skin thrown over his shoulder. The head was on the skin and its open mouth showed a fake red tongue and ugly, realistic-looking white fangs. Every night Tex ordered a drink, took a long swig, and threw the rest of it nonchalantly against the wall before proceeding to tell his latest batch of stories. His mouth was filthy. I'd heard rough language but nothing to equal his. One night I lit into him and chewed him out for using his tongue like that.

When I was through, Tex stood up, looking real black at me. Without more ado, he threw his leopard skin over my shoulder and yelled, "Man, you're the first fellow that's ever whipped me!"

Another night I saw a woman hit a cop over the head with her purse. He went down like a chunk of beef but came to his senses and threw her out bodily after that.

In the fall when the nights were getting cool, I watched two sailors of Mexican descent having a knife fight, outside the Sunshine Tavern. A knife fight is not quick like boxing, but slow, very slow. I saw the blade gleam, and sucked in my breath when one sailor groaned and fell to the ground. The cops came and dragged him away and the owner of the Sunshine Tavern emerged and threw a pail of water over the bloody sidewalk.

Sometimes I was asked to provide music at the different places, so I'd get up a four-piece band, usually with the Duchess as my pianist. For a long time I'd known I wanted music as a career. This was the way you had to break in to make it big. Or was it? I wasn't sure.

The sleazy vaudeville actors thought they were great stuff, but any smart person could see how lousy they were. Off key a good part of the time, cheap, vulgar.

I found myself shooting the breeze with anyone who came to sit at my table . . . drunks, prostitutes, queers. I was searching for something and not finding it. Reality? Life? Meaning? What was I looking for? I didn't know. I had a girl friend of sorts, a neighbor girl named Francie who came in to chat and make coffee for me each morning, and smooch; but she turned out to be married. Her husband was overseas and she was lonely.

In November I went down a second time to apply at the shipyards. The newspapers said they were desperate for help, but no dice. They turned me away. Floyd was in the Admiralty Islands, and his wife and baby in Minnesota. Mom read each letter out loud when it came. One of my former saxophone players wrote me a brief note from South Dakota to let me know that Shorty Long had been killed in action. Shorty . . . my piano player, gentle quiet Shorty. I found it hard to believe. His music was gone forever from the earth.

We hadn't heard from Jack for ages. Mom stewed about it. At Christmas we put up a little tree with colored lights, just for the three of us.

"I saved enough ration stamps for a small roast," said Mom. "But it doesn't seem much like a holiday with Floyd so far off and us miles from any relatives." She sniffed and stared out the window at a sailor walking down the street. The sight of him set her off again: "If only Jack were here, I'd feel a sight better . . . my sakes alive, that *is* Jack, isn't it?"

It was! With shouts of joy, we pummeled each other.

"They made me take another eye exam when I was almost through bootcamp," Jack told us grinning. "One I hadn't

134

memorized. They discovered I was blind in one eye. Guess I'll get on at the shipyard with you, Dad.''

Instead, when Christmas was over, he joined the city police force, passing every test with flying colors. It didn't matter about his eye. Their ranks depleted by war, they were hard up for strong, reliable men and were glad to get him.

The shipyards couldn't use me, the armed forces couldn't use me . . . at eighteen I looked old enough to fool people into thinking I was twenty-one, but I still couldn't support myself. I was dependent on Mom and Dad for that. For a little while I worked at a place where they gave out ration stamps. But I made up my own rules, since theirs were so rigid. If an old person had made an error with his stamps, why not slip him an extra book? Was it fair to cut meat or sugar completely out of his diet for several months because he was old and feeble and had made a mistake? The ration board didn't see things my way. They fired me.

How could I achieve a sense of worth? Playing my horn every now and then for a tawdry crowd, most of whom didn't know a thing about real music—that didn't do it. Life brought new questions all the time and I found no answers.

The bitterness of my hospital experiences had remained with me. God, at least the kind of God most people talked about, was a mockery. I could not discuss the matter with my parents. They led a full life. They did not know this emptiness.

Dad was not a religious man, yet he possessed a sense of well-being. He had a function on earth, a place, he was not afraid of change, he welcomed the variety it brought and with each change he achieved a new level of satisfaction. He had a sense of worth. In his way, my father seemed as puritanical as my mother, only Work was the God he worshipped.

Seldom did he speak of the meaning of life. He could pass the entire subject off with a wink: ''That's the Missus' department. She's got the whole thing figured out.''

Mom did, that's a fact. She didn't have to depend on a

preacher or anyone else. Through the years she'd found her answers in her Bible. Now she had mellowed enough to admit it wasn't all there, either. She found she could twist a phrase or two to make it fit her life.

Take smoking. After all, she commented mildly, the Bible didn't say it was right or wrong. It didn't mention smoking any place, so that must mean a person was supposed to decide for himself what he would do about it.

Jack, dignified in his brass-buttoned uniform, had found himself a sweetheart named Laurie. Overcome with shyness, he hid the fact from me for a few months, knowing how I would tease. He couldn't fool me though. Hadn't I seen them holding each other close in the shadows near our doorway when I came in at night? After I rounded a corner and caught them redhanded, Jack introduced me to her. Blushing, he admitted the date of the wedding was already set.

Yellow roses . . . yellow roses . . . In the mornings I lay in bed, watching the sunlight dance upon my wall. Then, for days on end, the spring rains ribboned past my window. I wondered how things would pan out for me. Would I ever become a musician with my name in colored lights? Would I some day have a wife, a family of my own? Later, after Mom and Dad and Jack had left for work, Francie knocked on the door and came in.

"Hello, Don. You want coffee? See, I brought sweet rolls from Brady's bakery. They're warm yet, smell!"

For a while we munched and chatted, then with a long sigh, she moved closer and let me cup my hand over her breast and unbutton the top part of her blouse and kiss her. Desire warmed me. I ached, filled with a terrible longing, but Francie pulled me away abruptly and whispered, "No . . . I can't . . . no . . . no . . . please, Don."

After she was gone, I wheeled down to the Blue Lion and got plastered. But it didn't help.

*nine*

---

"**Y**OU gotta see these cabins. They're swanky. You'll never regret it. We'll go in on the deal together and you can stay down in Seaside to manage 'em for me."

Dad had taken sick in the winter. The job at the shipyard was physically taxing for a man pushing sixty. He had to be on his feet, doing the same thing over and over for eight hours with short breaks to catch a cigarette or swill down a cup of coffee.

Tuckered out, he felt the lure of a new job in a different place. He was not easily swayed. But once he turned his mind in a particular direction, nobody could talk him out of it.

He sat out on the steps, listening to Henry Cleveland rave about this bunch of cabins. The more he heard, the better it sounded. Mom had come outside to get in on the conversation. Henry was a neighbor they'd known ever since we moved to Portland. They trusted his opinion.

"Seaside you say? Where's that?"

Henry cast an incredulous look at her. "You been in Oregon a whole year and don't know Seaside?"

Mom sounded vague. "It's over on the coast, isn't it?"

"Sure it's on the coast. It's a summer resort, teeming with activity. Has both an army and a naval base close to it . . . why the place is booming. My friend Carl was saying to me the other day he'd never seen such a booming town and I sez, Carl, you know you got something there. . . ."

"A change would be good for Kirk's health," Mom interrupted. "He's no spring chicken. And a small town does sound like it's what we want."

"Think of what this would mean to your son. Why it would give Don a way to support hisself if anything . . . an accident . . . happened to take both of you at once. Not that a body expects it but . . . oh you know what I mean."

"Is there money in it?" asked Dad.

"Tourist cabins? Money? You ain't kiddin' there's money . . . in a resort like Seaside? I'll say! I don't understand how come you folks never been over to the coast."

"You can't take a wheelchair on sand," Mom told him shortly. "It sinks in and won't budge. For a wheelchair, sand is as bad as gumbo."

Henry radiated triumph. "That's another thing . . . there's a cement promenade down in Seaside. Runs from one end of town to the other. Don'll be able to wheel along and enjoy the ocean without touching sand. That town's made for him."

"You think it's like he says it is?" Mom asked Dad that night.

"Of course. He wouldn't lie would he?"

Dad was so honest himself, he was unable to mistrust another man. The following week he quit his job at the shipyard. We drove to the coast and rented a cottage. Henry had promised to meet us the very next day.

After supper, Mom and Dad walked with me on the promenade, stopping often to watch the waves roll in and pound the shore. Overhead, gulls wheeled. To me, their cry sounded as haunting as the whistle of the night train I'd heard as a kid in Woonsocket, South Dakota.

A breeze blew off the water. I touched my tongue to my lips and tasted the salt.

"Look! A boat on the horizon . . ."Dad pointed. "Probably a victory ship. "And see the fishing vessel?"

Children dotted the sand, building castles, digging holes to trap the incoming tide. The beach was by no means crowded, yet a number of soldiers and sailors sprawled here and there on blankets, making love to their girls. One family was busy cooking wieners over a driftwood fire. Farther down the beach, a group of high school boys had a softball game going.

The sea shimmered violet and green in the dusk and the sky looked iridescent, like the inside of a shell. I could hear the squeak of a harmonica playing a popular wartime hit . . . "When the lights go on again all over the world."

Servicemen strolled on the promenade with buddies or with their sweethearts. I noticed several MPs and SPs patrolling the area. The promenade skirted a rise and when you looked toward town you could see a sea of white hats, the town was that full of sailors.

As I wheeled, I picked up snatches of conversation.

"Whadja tell me yer name is . . . Jeanie? Jeanie, lets you and me go for a ride on the ferris wheel."

"Hey Jim, I gotta five spot I can blow in town. We can find ourselves a coupla broads and take in the show at the Monterey Club. . . ."

It grew darker. The sky throbbed with stars. We walked and looked and listened.

At last Mom said, "I'm tired and Henry'll be down early in the morning to see to our cabins. Let's go back to the cottage."

The cabins. They were a great idea. Anyone could tell that at first glance. Good-looking cabins in A-one condition. A fine investment.

139

But . . . Henry shook his head sadly after we'd looked them over and talked to the real estate agent. "I just don't have *that* much money to spend. Hang on, Kirkendall, we'll look around a little more."

He'd gotten Dad to give up perfectly good wages at the shipyard, dragged him down here to invest in tourist cabins . . . and now no cabins?

"He's some friend!" I muttered when he'd gone away.

"I trust Henry," Dad told me. "He'll find something. I know he will."

Pretty soon he did come up with a new idea. Dad heard him out, weighed the matter in his own mind, and fell for it.

"What are you signing?" I demanded when I wheeled in and saw the papers spread over the kitchen table in the cottage.

"What'd I tell you?" Dad looked elated. "Instead of tourist cabins we've decided to invest in . . ."

"Invest in what?"

"Oyster beds."

*"Oyster beds? Are you serious?"*

"Yup. Of course I'm serious. It's a real industry down here on the coast and . . ."

Shades of the Drake Estate! I didn't dare say it out loud. I was certain Dad had those Drake Estate papers around somewhere yet. But this Henry Cleveland was beginning to make old Oscar Hartzell look like a Christmas card cherub.

"Look Dad, do me a favor. Don't write a check until we find out more about these . . . these oyster beds."

He kept on writing.

"Dad!" I was pleading now. "Please Dad, listen! Damn it, listen! I don't think you can buy land that's under the ocean. It doesn't make sense. Ask somebody who knows more about it than your friend Henry."

"All right, Don," he agreed finally. "I'm willing to wait. We've got enough to live on for another few weeks."

Days passed. Henry looked at a whole series of cabins up

140

for sale but discovered none to suit his pocketbook. He never mentioned oyster beds again. Meanwhile, he was a constant visitor at our house. He was growing fat off Mom's cooking, he took time to get a tan on the beach, he spoke importantly about the deals he'd made and those he was about to make.

"Don't you put down cash on anything he offers," I warned Dad. Maybe he wasn't getting sick of Henry but I was. Before long I found a solution.

"Dad . . . you want to know where a guy can really pull in money?"

"Where?"

"Concessions. I've been watching the fellows that run 'em. There's one in particular . . . the bottle ball game. I saw the wad of bills the man had at the end of the day. And the place is up for sale. It would be a good buy, Dad."

By this time he was tired of sitting around. He hot-footed it down to talk to the owner of the bottle ball game. He asked questions, he took in the soldiers and sailors, tourists and children streaming in and out of the other concessions, and then he said quietly, "I can give you a thousand dollars down."

The place was ours. We were concessionaires!

"What I was aiming to do," I confided to Laurie and Jack who brought their baby down for a weekend visit, "was to tie up Dad's money so it wasn't handy for old Henry any more. That skunk! It worked, too!"

"Come on everybody, come on in and try your luck at bottle ball. Three balls for two bits. The game's easy. Win a kewpie doll, win a silver cup, win a blanket or a china teapot . . . we got the best prizes going . . . you can see for yourself we do, come on in everybody and have a go at it."

Our bottle ball game was in a good location, across the street from the Monterey Club, in the heart of town. People came. Old, young, fat, thin, beautiful, ugly people. From servicemen to sunburned, mosquito-bitten, skinny-legged kids, they came.

"I gotta have that Kewpie doll . . . the one with the baby

blue sash on it," sighed a chunky lady in a cheap cotton sun dress. "Willyum, you hear me? I gotta have that Kewpie doll."

"Jeez, Ella Mae, like I was tellin ya . . . this beach ain't nothin to Coney Island!"

"Hey kid, gimme a dollar's worth of balls so I can win sumpin' good for my honey to take home."

The damp air smelled of sunlight and salt and buttered popcorn. In the evenings, whenever the door of the Monterey Club swung open, I could hear the band. One of these days I'd get up a trio and play my horn again. At the moment, I concentrated on being a barker, the best durn barker for miles around.

"Step right up, ladies and gents, and have a try. Bottle ball is easy. No tricks, no skill. Anyone can do it, so help yourself." Of course there was a trick, but never mind about that. It was all in the way you set up the wooden bottles. When you set them close together, a good pitcher could knock them down without a miss every time. We soon picked out the pros and were careful to set their bottles slightly apart so it would be impossible to get a strike.

The concessionaire's life was separate from the life of the tourists. We worked hard until two or three in the morning, then closed shop and joined the rest of the crowd at the steakhouse to eat and smoke and trade stories about some of the nutty tourists we'd run across during the day.

"This dumb blond named Mabel . . . every day she comes to shoot darts at balloons. Has her heart set on that giant tiger I got on the shelf. Gotta duck when she shoots, man. She's that bad!"

"Have you run across old Frank? Claims he's gonna be a hundred and three next March. Ain't nobody smarter than old Frank."

We found a camaraderie, a feeling of good will. If you needed money, someone would loan it to you. If you got into trouble, somebody would be on hand to bail you out. If you mentioned a sick daughter or a wife with a miscarriage, you could be sure of a sympathetic ear at any hour of the day or night. If you needed a lift to Portland to pick up a load of prizes at the concessionaire store, no problem. We laughed together, wept together, worked and played together and banded with one another to squeeze money out of the tourists so we could live through the winter when things got quiet around Seaside.

But, during the war, things never did get too quiet. After the tourists went home in the fall, plenty of soldiers and sailors were left. I became buddies with many of them. We went out for drinks in the different clubs around Astoria and Seaside. I sensed their longing. It was wartime . . . they had their girl friends . . . but in war, when the Navy says you got to move on, you got to move on, brother. So why not do it now . . . what harm? I saw many things . . . a leg sticking out of a telephone booth, two bodies clinging to one another in the sand. I heard voices in the night when I came out of the bottle ball game ready for a hamburger. It was war and you gotta do what you gotta do. You might never have another chance.

I looked at the soldiers and sailors and I thought about Floyd, wondering how he was doing in the Admiralty Islands, and I thought about his wife back home. It was a long hard wait for both of them.

Young people my age came to throw balls at the wooden bottles and stayed to talk. I made friends with a cleancut blond fellow who drove a Cadillac, a high school senior named Bob Sealy. Bob's family owned a summer house, an ostentatious home designed like the fo'c's'le of a ship, with a view of the ocean.

"You play anything?" I asked when he paused in the middle of his bottle ball game to listen to the music pouring out of the Monterey Club.

"You bet I do. Drums. How about you?"

"Trumpet. We should get together some time."

"You met Norton here?" asked Bob on another night. The kid he had in tow was fat, friendly, easy to talk to. He played the yukelele but was interested in learning guitar.

I'd found myself some buddies who talked my language . . . music. From that time on, we were a threesome.

"See if your folks can manage a couple of hours without you," suggested Bob when he stopped by on a slow afternoon. "I'd like to take you up to my house to hear my drums."

I hesitated. Clearly, he'd forgotten about my wheelchair.

When I mentioned steps, he dismissed the idea with nonchalance. "No trouble. We'll pack you in."

That was the beginning of many good times. Bob didn't fool around with drums, he played them. He had real talent.

First thing he did after packing me into the house was to pull open the living room drapes to show me the ocean. I drank in the scene. I was impressed by the magnificent view and impressed, too, by the grand piano. It made me think of Shorty Long and the times we'd had together. I knew I wanted to be making music again.

I visited often in Bob's home. Mama Sealy got along famously with me. Carefully coiffured and fashionably dressed, she overlooked the enormous gap between her financial circumstances and mine and set me at ease.

It wasn't long before I talked Norton into discarding his yukelele and buying a guitar. With his musical brilliance, he became adept at the instrument. Now we could play around in different clubs as a trio whenever we got asked. To my delight one night we ran into my old friend, the Duchess, playing honky-tonk piano in a bar in Astoria.

Our concession had proved so successful that when the penny pitch went up for sale, Dad bought it, and the shuffleboard game too. It took the three of us to run the concessions but when one of us wanted a night off, we hired a kid to come in and take over for us.

I had a favorite small restaurant where I liked to hang out. The waitresses were friendly and the service good. One of them, Beth, knew exactly how well done I wanted my hamburger . . . just that much and no more, and how I liked my coffee.

Beth was a cute trick, petite, alive. Whenever she caught a glimpse of me at the corner table, she'd do her best to get a coffee break so she could sit and talk awhile. I found out she loved to dance and swim and she'd seen most of the current movies. One night when a new Hepburn and Tracy came to town I asked her to go with me after work.

I had a date! I had a date with a cute little waitress who could have winked her eye and gone out with any soldier or sailor in town.

After that whenever I asked her she said yes. Yes, yes, yes! A girl was saying yes to me!

"Why?"

She laughed. "What do you mean, why? You're unique."

On warm days we picnicked at Cullaby Lake. Sometimes with Bob or Norton, sometimes with Tommy, a sailor friend of mine and his wife. Those times one of the fellows packed me from the car to the shore.

I had a girl who laughed at me and admired me and wanted to be my sweetheart. No doubt she'd broken the heart of many another guy . . . hadn't I seen her dancing at the Sand Castle and the Monterey, looking coquettishly into their eyes and snuggling close?

We sat outside in the dark, talking about a million things . . . where we wanted to go and what we'd do when we got there. We were human, we kissed and then we fought. Arguments . . . in the end, what are they about? Differences of opinion, hurt feelings without meaning to hurt, and then more kisses, delicious on the tongue, to make up.

One night when I went over to the restaurant for coffee, she looked piqued. She slumped into the chair beside me, leaning under the table to shuck off her shoes.

"There." She sighed. "Don, I don't know what to do. My landlord's raising the rent. I can't pay any more than what I'm paying now."

"S'pose you threaten to move out. Would he let you be?"

145

"Not him. The old skinflint. But I only wait tables four nights a week. That's not enough money . . .''

"I bet Mom and Dad would rent you our spare room. It's on the ground floor, off the kitchen. I know they wouldn't charge as much as you're paying now."

She looked over at me with a radiant face. "Would you mind asking? It would be a help. Tell your mother I'd be glad to do some of her cleaning and cooking."

"Of course," Mom agreed the minute I asked.

"I can be free an hour or two to lend a hand moving her gear on Saturday if she wants," added Dad.

And so Beth moved into our spare room. I lay in bed, thinking about it, on Saturday night. I could hear her opening and closing drawers, putting sweaters and other stuff away. Mom and Dad had turned in early. The house was quiet.

I wondered if Beth might like to help out in the bottle ball game during the afternoon before she went to work. She seemed to be hard up for cash. I made up my mind to ask her, first thing in the morning. She must have gone to bed. I could no longer hear any sounds in the other room.

I liked to lie there in the quiet house long after the folks had gone to sleep, and read. Tonight I was so engrossed in my book, I did not hear my bedroom door crack open. I glanced up, surprised, when I heard Beth's voice.

"Donald? I saw your light on. I couldn't sleep."

Like a blythe and winsome child, she crawled in beside me and pulled up the covers.

To succeed in making love! I had proved I could do it and it was a tremendous boost to my ego. I suspected Dad had known all along that I'd be able to do so one day . . . hadn't he continually badgered me to go out and find myself a girl?

I had thought about it many times . . . what I would do if I found I could not make love in a normal way. Each time I'd brushed the question aside, knowing I'd find a way to deal

146

with it when the time came. Other people had found ways to work through such a difficult problem, hadn't they?

After that first night, I felt very possessive with Beth, jealous when she so much as flirted with a customer or stopped to pass the time of day with an old sailor friend. She was my girl and I expected her to do everything with me. But, as the weeks flew by, I realized she wanted to be able to keep her old friends too.

One day as I wheeled by a restaurant I looked through the window and, sure enough, there she was, having coffee with another fellow.

Angrily I wheeled in to the table. "What the hell do you think you're doing?"

"I've got a perfect right to be in here with whoever I please," she retorted. She made a saucy face. "You can't stop me."

"Like hell I can't!"

All the way home to the cottage I fumed. That night as soon as she got home she went to her bedroom. I heard her rummaging around, packing her suitcase. When she left I made no attempt to stop her.

In a few days, after my temper cooled, I dropped by the restaurant where she worked.

"Beth?" asked one of the other waitresses. "Didn't she tell you? She's taken a job in Astoria."

Maybe she wanted me to come after her but I wasn't about to do that. I turned my mind to other matters.

For a long time I'd had my eye on the photo shop. A small shop with a thriving business because of the wartime boom. Kids, adults, servicemen, sweethearts poured in and out of the place to buy pictures to send off in letters, to carry in wallets, to set on the kitchen windowsill or slip under a pillow at night.

I watched and waited. I had no cash of my own to buy such a shop. Dad and Mom and I were in business together. I had no special needs, but when it came to buying a shop of my own, I was not, at the moment, independent enough to do it.

An unexpected thing happened. A state rehabilitation counselor, combing the area because of war veterans, noticed me in my wheelchair and stopped to pass the time of day.

"You can't count me as a shut-in," I teased him. "And handicapped? I bet I can do anything you can do and maybe a few things you can't." I wasn't considering minor difficulties like steps.

"Can you drive?" he tested me.

"Not now, but I will some day. I once rode in a car with hand controls. When I get enough money I'll have one."

In turn, I tested him. "How about you . . . can you play the trumpet?"

"No," he had to admit with a laugh. "I guess I *am* handicapped in that respect. But can you?"

"Sure can. I've had my own nine-piece band. Right now I play the horn sometimes at the Monterey and around in other clubs."

He looked slightly nonplussed. "You mentioned money. Did you know the state is willing to take a gamble and set you up in business for yourself?"

"Great!" I shouted. "I wish I'd known that sooner. How about the photo shop down on the main drag? The owner's getting ready to move. Would the state help me buy it?"

"They wouldn't help you buy it," he said quietly. "They'd pay for the whole darn thing, taking the risk that you'll make a go of it. Interested?"

Interested? Of course I was! Before the month was out, I had my own business. The counselor and I were fast friends. I noticed he deleted the word *handicapped* from his vocabulary in my presence.

Over coffee, we talked.

"The state will pay the cost of any course you want to take, too," he told me. "Courses having to do with earning a livelihood . . . bookkeeping, typing, business ed, not courses in the aesthetic field."

148

"How about radio announcing? I've always wanted to go on the air."

He smiled. "You've got the voice for it. But radio would come in the category of aesthetics . . . drama, the art world."

"Aw come on. If you worked at it, I bet you could get me some on-the-spot training. You have pull, don't you?"

He realized I was serious. The following day he drove over to have a talk with the owner of the KAST radio station in Astoria.

"What did he say?" I asked as soon as I saw the counselor again.

"He didn't say yes and he didn't say no. He sent you a message. He said, 'Tell that guy if he can sell his own spot on radio, I'll let him have half an hour.' "

Two days passed before I could take time out from my photo shop to do what I had in mind. The third night, when Mom was able to take over for an hour, the owner of the Monterey Club wasn't in. The fourth night I found him.

I told him about the bands I'd had in South Dakota and said, "I could double your patronage at the Monterey if I put you on the air for half an hour every evening. It would be well worth buying the time. I wouldn't need to do a thing except be master of ceremonies . . . interview clients, tell a joke or two . . . I'm pretty quick at ad libbing."

"Sounds good to me," he answered. "You're on. I'll call KAST and let 'em know."

The program was a wild success. I wore earphones and looked official. I wheeled around to the different tables and talked to homesick servicemen. I cracked jokes. I pulled them out of the doldrums, I flattered them, I teased them, I was a hit.

"Hey fella, that's some sweetheart you got. Quite a dish!"

"You say you're from Texas? And your buddy here hails from Arkansas? What's your favorite hit? I'll get the band to play it."

There was a magic about being on the air.

Everyone wanted to have a turn at the mike so their buddies on the base could hear them. They wanted to write back home and say "Hey Mom, Dad . . . I got interviewed."

I packed them into the Monterey Club. Because I was MC, scores of people recognized me and greeted me on the street. The minute they heard me speak, they'd say, "Aren't you Don Kirkendall, the guy that's on the air about ten o'clock each night? Sure you are!"

Sailors stopped by to play bottle ball or to have their pictures taken at the photo shop and grinned when they saw me. "I know you . . . I was there last night, didja see me? I'll try to get back tonight."

Just before I went off the air one night a phone call came in. I finished up the program and rolled over to the desk to answer it. It was Beth.

"Oh Don, I can't believe it! I turned on the radio when I got home to the apartment tonight and heard you." She laughed. "I thought you must be down at the station here in Astoria, so I called KAST. Their technician put me through to you."

"I've got to go back and work at my photo shop," I told her. "But I'll get Mom or Dad to take over tomorrow night. You want to meet me at the Club? I go off the air at ten-thirty."

"It's a date. I'll be there."

After the show she looked me over with sparkling eyes. "This is so good for you! This and the photo shop. How long have you been running it? Are you making money on it? Do you like it?"

When she'd run down and we'd talked a bit, she flashed me one of her old grins and said, "I hate the place I'm at. I'm moving back to Seaside . . . they're looking for a counter girl at Jolly's Dinette."

"In that case, how about a show on Saturday night?"

The old rift was mended. Like that.

As soon as they'd graduated from high school, Bob Sealy and Norton had joined the armed forces. It had meant the disbanding of our threesome, temporarily at least. Sometimes I visited with Mama Sealy. We talked about those summer afternoons when her living room had vibrated with music and laughter.

"At least you're not lonely," she said with a wink. "I see Beth is back in town. And you have your photo shop and the job at the Monterey to keep you out of mischief."

I'd been working at the Monterey for nearly half a year. The live broadcast had continued to be such a success that the club overflowed almost every night of the week. A change would have to be made. The owner of the place saw that and I did too.

"It's a fire hazard, Don. Besides, the waitresses can't get through the mob to serve customers. I think we'll have to stop the program. I'm sorry. I liked it. It was good."

I thought of a way to continue with radio. Why not direct a music and talk program from the station at Astoria through a studio of my own each afternoon? I got a friend to give me a lift over to KAST so I could talk to the owner.

"Your broadcast from the Monterey has been tops," was his answer. "As long as you can make this show pay for itself, you're on. Better get busy and find some customers."

It wasn't long before I'd fixed up a small studio with table, chairs, mike, and headphones. The Monterey bought advertising time and so did a local furniture store and a beauty parlor. I wheeled down to Jolly's Dinette to tell Beth the news.

"You'll be a disk jockey with your own show? And a studio?" I knew she was impressed.

In my heart I knew that was the real reason she wanted to be my girl . . . she thought I was good-looking, a snappy dresser, a clever conversationalist. To her, being a disk jockey was no small thing . . . it was a glamorous job. Did she actually love me? She wanted to be with me, that much was obvious. As far as I was concerned, I did love her and I felt I could make her happy.

151

*ten*

———————————————

W HEN I'd earned enough money, I bought an engagement ring. Beth drew back, reluctant to let me slip it over her
finger.

"Come on, Beth. You know you want it."

"It's beautiful. But I like my freedom. I'm not ready to be
tied to any man."

"Oh yes you are!"

"Maybe . . ." Laughing, she accepted the diamond ring,
twisting it in the light to admire it. "Thank you," she whispered
as she gave me a kiss. "You're sweet, Donald."

Six weeks later we were married. Mom and Dad were happy
to let us stay on at their cottage. I was not earning enough to
support a wife. It didn't embarrass me . . . not at first. My parents
and I had worked out this satisfactory arrangement with money
and work. They didn't tinker with my studio. The radio job was
mine alone. But they helped run the photo shop and I helped with
the bottle ball game, and we shared our earnings.

But how do you share a marriage with your mother and father? And how, as man and wife, do you find a place alone when someone is always in the next room? It had not been easy to find privacy when I was twenty-three and single, but I soon found marriage increased the difficulty.

It was the summer of 1945. In August the war ended. When the announcement came over the radio, the entire town of Seaside went wild. People yelled like maniacs and cheered and jumped up and down. Horns honked. Strangers kissed each other. Soldiers and sailors let out whoops of joy. Many wept.

"Thank God!" Mom kept saying over and over again. "Thank God! I suppose Floyd will be coming home soon."

Mom was particularly fond of Floyd. There had always been that special bond of mother and firstborn son.

Seaside would change with the end of the war. But how long would it take? What would happen when the armed forces began to muster out? No one could predict. I couldn't envision a Seaside without hundreds of men in uniform. At least half of my photo shop business came from soldiers and sailors wanting to have pictures taken . . . pictures to carry in wallets, pictures to send to sweethearts miles away. Much of the crowd in the Monterey Club and in the different taverns was made up of men from the army and naval bases, too.

It wouldn't happen all at once. The process would be slow but inevitable. I put the idea out of my head because I had something else to worry about. I had been married for two and a half months and now Beth wanted a divorce.

"Why?" I pleaded. "Tell me why?"

Our lives didn't mesh, she pointed out. There were things we couldn't share . . . dancing . . . swimming. But mainly she just didn't want to be married to me anymore. And she didn't want to discuss it further.

"You've got no real grounds for divorce," I argued. "What if I won't give it to you?"

"Then I guess I'll have to wait."

We'd talked back and forth about it several times. But this time the look in her eye told me she was serious.

She climbed into bed with me as usual that night. When I awoke in the morning the bed beside me was empty.

She did not come back.

It hit hard, that break. My pride was wounded. What good was a man who couldn't earn a real living or hang onto a girl like Beth? A no-good phony bum, that's what I was. Someone who messed around with a photo shop and a half-hour radio program . . . and played the horn now and then at dances. But so what?

Badly shaken, I floundered through each day, dreading the thought another one would come. I was lonely for Beth. I wanted Beth. But Beth was gone.

I got word she'd left for a job in Juneau, Alaska. Shortly after that I lost my radio show. Not enough merchants were buying advertising time.

When I went to the Monterey at night I took my own bottle of Scotch. I could hold my liquor well, disguising the fact I was looped whenever I was asked to play my trumpet. Nobody else knew. But I knew. I hated myself.

One night I downed drink after drink, unable to obliterate the darkness raging inside me. In a drunken fit of self-pity, I managed to get home. I grabbed a bottle of sleeping pills from the bathroom cupboard. How many did I take? I didn't bother to count. I didn't care.

The combination of Scotch and sedatives had a lethal effect. I found what I'd been seeking . . . oblivion. The next thing I knew, the emergency truck from the fire department was at our door. I was having my stomach pumped out.

When the ordeal was over, I lay there exhausted.

"Donald . . . " whispered my mother. "Oh Donald!"

I heard another sound. I opened my eyes and saw my father weeping. Never to my knowledge had he done this before. No tears when he had carried me home from the hospital paralyzed by polio. No tears when his father died or the day we buried his mother. None when Floyd and Jack went off to war and he wondered if he would ever see either of them again.

A flood of remorse swept over me. I wanted to comfort him but could find no words. It came to me, in an instant, how much my parents had done for me through the years, and how they had cared . . . and what grief I was causing them.

Something happened to me then, a turning.

The following night I wheeled into the Monterey. When the waitress stopped at my table, I turned my empty bottle of Scotch upside down and said, "Gimme coffee tonight, Dolly."

"You sick or something?"

"No. I mean it."

"Listen, Donald Kirkendall, I know you . . ."

"Look, I'm not fooling around. I'm through with booze. At least with hard liquor. I'm done, I tell you. The only thing I want is some coffee."

It was a long time before I could bring myself to take even the smallest nip of Scotch again.

I became determined to lick those blue moods. A thought flashed through my mind. This was a decision like that childish choice in the hospital many years ago—"I'll take jelly."

It was simply that. A decision.

Fortunately, I had a host of friends, young and old, surrounding me. Both Sealy and Norton were back in Seaside. And there were countless others. A whole town full of people I knew and loved. A favorite of mine was Ernie the Greek who ran a fine restaurant.

Ernie liked to give me a hard time. As soon as my wheelchair appeared in the doorway of his establishment, he would come at me with a meat cleaver, calling out oaths and insults while those clients who did not know him gasped. Brandishing the cleaver, he continued to yell until he reached me. Then with a sudden

155

change of heart, he'd throw his brawny arm around my shoulders and give me a warm greeting. This was a regular act. He never missed a time.

I could always get cheered up at Ernie's. One look at my face would tell him how I felt, that I needed companionship, so he'd settle down and regale me with tales of his son Alex. Alex had been a friend of mine for a long time. A thin fellow with dusky skin and a long nose and curly hair, he'd come in often to play bottle ball and to chat, maybe to take me for a ride in his car. Like other boys, he'd gone away to war.

I felt sick inside the day Ernie greeted me with reddened eyes and informed me that Alex had come down with polio while in the service. Of course he knew that was how I had ended up in a wheelchair. It was the only thing he could think of—Alex, his pride and his joy!

One day when I stopped by the restaurant Ernie looked as if he would burst with news. Alex had begun to recover. Soon he would be home for a visit!

"He says he is in a wheelchair most of the time. But he is beginning to take steps."

As soon as he hit town, Alex wheeled over to visit me. We talked for a long time. He looked very thin. And it was obvious he was weak. But he got out of his chair for a few minutes and showed me how he could shuffle slowly across the room.

"The doctor at the vets' hospital says I'll really walk again, perhaps with only a small limp." Happy, he smiled. We compared wheelchairs then. Josephine was holding up remarkably well, but today I was using an inexpensive folding chair I'd owned for a while. Alex's chair folded too, but was far superior in design and quality. He made me slide into it and try it out.

We talked of many things, what he would study when he got out of service, and what he wanted to do.

Late in the afternoon he rose. "I promised my father I'd be back at five."

156

"Hey, that's my wheelchair you've got," I said quickly when he sat down in the wrong one.

He rolled over to the door before turning to answer.

"Why so it is. I don't suppose the army will ever know the difference, do you?" And out he went in the cheap folding chair, leaving the good one as a parting gift for me.

As more and more men mustered out of the service, business at the concessions in Seaside lessened. The bottle ball game continued to be popular so Dad kept that one concession open. I sold my photo shop. Mom started to work in a dress shop down the street, adjacent to the town's ballroom. In a few months she decided to buy it. She wrote to her sister Maud, my Uncle Harry's wife in Minnesota, and borrowed the money.

I found a new source of income. With the assistance of Sealy and Norton, I started a *Shopping News*. From the beginning, the merchants in town seemed interested. Many of them bought advertising space. I had not lost my knack at drawing so I did the cartoons sprinkled throughout the pages. I designed every ad, Sealy did the typing, and Norton and I took turns writing editorials.

I saved my earnings to buy a car. Mom and Dad never said a word, but Jack, when he and Laurie were visiting, told me he thought it was a waste of money.

"Seventy-five dollars for that old thing? A four-door Chevvy sedan cut down into a pick up? What the hell do you want a car for when you can't drive it?"

"Thanks for your brotherly opinion. But I do want it. Maybe I can't drive it but other guys can."

A car of my own would give me some degree of independence. I could pay for the gas and the upkeep. With someone else at the wheel, I could make the rounds to collect advertising customers for the *Shopping News*.

Like my old wheelchair, my cutdown Chevvy pick up had a name. I christened her Cora. Cora had stood idle for years. She was, as Jack had pointed out, a cheap, broken-down old car.

During the next weeks, with the coaching of mechanically minded friends, I learned everything there was to know about a car. I learned about brakes, tie rods, mufflers, carburetors, wiring, heaters, headlights, radiators, valves, and clutches. It was a proud day when Cora decided to run.

In addition to a car, I had found myself a new sweetheart, a flashy redhead named Lollie. Lollie was more cosmopolitan than Beth. She'd had a job in Chicago, she had been married and divorced, she had a baby boy. Right now she and her sister were running a restaurant on the edge of town.

The Seaside winters were long and there wasn't much to do. Often a gang of us would drive out to Lollie's restaurant for coffee and hamburgers. One of the boys began to date Lollie's sister and, at the same time, I found myself asking Lollie if she'd like to take in a show.

And so a new relationship began. I seemed to be developing a bad habit. I was falling in love with every girl I went with! Lollie flattered me and gave me a good feeling about myself. She was having financial troubles with her restaurant. I had a small amount of savings in a bank in Seaside so, feeling very masculine and needed, I helped her pay off her debts.

Once again, I wanted her to be all mine . . . no dating other fellows. Marriage seemed to be a sure way to fix this and besides, Lollie herself was eager to settle down. This time too, I made the mistake of attempting to have us live as man and wife, in my folks' cottage.

Before marriage, Lollie was fun. After the wedding, life became one long screaming fight. She wanted me to do this, she wanted me to do that. She wanted a whole wardrobe of pretty new clothes, and a modern apartment. She screamed and nagged.

I grew very fond of Joey, her one-and-a-half-year-old baby. But slowly and surely I realized this was one marriage that never should have been legalized in the first place. I held on for nine months. This time, after a particularly bitter quarrel, it was I who asked my wife to leave.

Perhaps I was not cut out to be a married man. I mulled the idea over and rejected it. Some day I wanted to have a wife and family. But, as I thought about Beth and Lollie, I had to be truthful with myself. I had not found the right girl yet.

Was it because I moved on wheels? Many times I stared down at my legs, flaccid, immobile on the footrests of my chair. No . . . in the worst moments, I could not use those legs to excuse myself from living. Beth and Lollie—a host of women—had preferred my company to that of other men. I had wit and originality, I had proved I could have an intimate relationship. Why then did I fail in marriage? Over and over I asked myself the question.

Sealy was smitten with a new girl friend. They would be married soon. Besides women and music, he had another passion . . . flying. He'd bought a plane, renting hangar space for it at the tiny airport on the outskirts of Seaside.

Through Bob I, too, became absorbed in flying. The naval air base near Astoria had been converted into a private airport. We hung around there and the Seaside field, discussing the assets of various aircraft and watching the planes take off and land. Bob loved to fly. Often he invited me to go with him.

For years I had dreamed of piloting a plane. Now I stubbornly began to look for a way. I talked to the owner of the Seaside airport.

"Tell you what," he suggested. "The government is paying for lessons for any GI returning to the area. We could work it this way, Don. Every time you bring in a GI to sign up for lessons, I'll let you have one yourself."

That should be easy! I had many friends returning from a stint in the service. And, too, I was not shy about approaching strangers.

Soon I was learning how to fly.

It was not the poetry of flying . . . the immensity of the view from the air, the feeling of soaring that pleased me most, but the risks I could take. Any of the risk-taking adventures so dear to the hearts of men were foreign experiences to me. Never

159

had I skiied or hiked a mountain trail or rappelled down a rock cliff or raced a car or played a game like polo or hockey.

The feeling of speed . . . that was the exhilarating feeling I loved. Often, to get a thrill, we flew low over the beach, pulled up until the plane stalled, and then did the necessary nose dive to gain air speed and get into control again.

Once when we spotted two girls riding horseback on the shore we flew down within fifty feet of the ground and buzzed them. The terrified horses took off but not until they'd dumped their riders upon the sand. That time, when we reached the airport, the owner had already received a nuisance call.

Coolly, he looked us in the eye. "Did you fellows happen to buzz a couple of girls on horseback a little while ago?"

"Who . . . us?"

"If I ever find out who did it," he warned, "somebody's gonna have their pilot's license pulled."

We were less daring after that. For a week or two, anyway.

One day Sealy came tearing over to the cottage. "Don, there's one plane in Astoria you've got to see. It's a beauty . . . a Grumman Goose. I came home to get you."

This amphibious plane had been fixed up in style, for use as a corporation plane. It was yellow and had the hatch on top. I was dubious.

"Jeez, how the hell do you think I can get into that, Sealy?"

"I'll pack you up the ladder."

I counted the steps. Seven up to the hatch, but then how many other steps down inside the plane?

"Don't worry about a thing. We'll make it. I want you to see the interior."

He hoisted me onto his back and started slowly up the steep ladder. I pictured what we must look like if anybody was around watching. A ridiculous sight. I couldn't help laughing.

Huffing and puffing, he got up to the hatch, shifted my weight, and started down.

160

"Hey, wait now . . . *we're stuck!*"

By now both of us were shaking with laughter. The hatch happened to be quite small and we were, indeed, stuck.

We struggled to work ourselves free and Bob got safely down the ladder and deposited me in one of the posh upholstered easy chairs with a long sigh of relief.

We sat there laughing until we had to wipe our eyes.

"For Pete's sake, you bloody bastard!" he exclaimed suddenly. "How'm I ever going to get you *out* of here?" The look of panic on his face sent me off into another gale of laughter.

By late October the tourists had boarded their summer houses and the beach was empty except for a solitary walker here and there. A heavy wind blew in off the ocean, scouring the rock jetties, rattling the window panes of our cottage. Coast guard warnings went out over the radio. A storm was on its way.

This one was wilder than many I'd seen. The tide was in and waves surged right over the promenade, sending rivulets of water gushing into the middle of town. When the rain subsided, Bob came and got me and we drove up as close as we could get to the shore to have a look. The ocean had been on the rampage for several days. The wind still had a vicious bite to it.

"I bet that's beautiful from the air," I told him.

"I bet it is. What're we waiting for?"

The danger of what we were about to do never entered our heads. We tore out to the airport. Nobody in sight. Somehow, Bob managed to get his plane out of the hangar alone. A Cessna with a 75 horse power engine, it could only carry the two of us. It rocked on its wheels as he prepared to hoist me in.

Into that strong wind we soared, veering toward the Tilamook Head. It wasn't long before both of us felt shaky inside. The wind buffeted the plane, creating a frightening noise like the pounding of many hammers on the wings. Something was making a crinkly, rattling sound, too, as if someone was shaking a bunch of sheet metal. Maybe the plane would blow to pieces in midair before we had a chance to get her down! I shot a look at Bob. He'd grown pale, too frightened to crack jokes anymore.

"We'll just take her over the lighthouse and back," he called out, trying to make himself heard above the wind. "That OK by you?"

"Sure thing." Neither of us wanted to let on how nervous we felt. During some moments in that roaring wind we were both holding onto the wheel to steady the plane.

Bob concentrated on bouncing the plane down on the small runway at Seaside. We caught our breath and sat a few moments without words.

"Well anyway," said Bob, "we made it. For a little while I wasn't sure we would."

The owner of the Seaside airport was a superb pilot. It annoyed him to hear the kind of risks some of the younger pilots and instructors were taking. I had logged many hours, although I'd never soloed. For a long time he had watched me flying, with someone else along, doing the daredevil stunts I loved to do.

One day before Steve, the friend who was with me, helped me out of the plane, the owner came out. "Stay right there, Don. I'm gonna take you up and show you 'zactly what this little plane can do. You . . . you . . . think you're so smart. You don't know it yet, but you're a fool!"

Eyes blazing, he lifted me back into the second seat and climbed into the cockpit. He took the plane into the air and proceeded to do the most dangerous stunts he could think to do. At times he flew so low over the ocean to skip waves that he was wetting our wheels. He skimmed over the beach, hopping logs, letting first one wheel hit the ground and then the other. He took the plane into a power-on stall by holding the wheel going up until it stalled in midair. Those times we gained terrific speed as we started down . . . such speed I was terrified we might nose dive into the sand, but adeptly the pilot pushed the wheel forward at the crucial moment and brought us out fast. By the time we rolled down the runway of the airport, I was trembling violently. One false move on the part of the pilot and both of us would have been dead.

"Jesus!" I muttered under my breath. "Oh Jesus." Out loud I said, "Thank you. I got the message."

Without a word he lifted me out.

I was but seven hours away from a license of my own. I knew the FAA would restrict me to soloing in one plane, an Ercoupe. This was the only plane available with the rudder control tied in from the rudder to the aileron so that it could be worked by hand. Thus far, I'd learned to fly without using the rudder control, by tipping the plane and allowing the rudder to follow the aileron.

For a long time I'd had a plan in mind to solve this problem by means of a simple invention. So simple, in fact, that I was surprised nobody else had thought of it. I drew up a sketch. In any airplane piloted by means of a stick instead of a wheel, a Silvair for instance, why not pass the rudder cable along the stick, put a wheel on the stick, and loop the rudder control over this wheel pulley fashion? You would have to cross the cables over each other so the wheel could be turned by hand for rudder control and the stick would function exactly as it had before.

Dad saw the point right away. "Take it down and show Inman, the owner of the field. You could get a patent on that, Don."

"The thing's so damn simple. He'll probably laugh at me."

"What the hell . . . show him anyway. It's good!"

As soon as he saw my plan, a look of real amazement crossed Inman's face. "I'll be jiggered! I never saw anything like it before and it's that simple! Do me a favor and apply for a patent, Don. I'm serious!"

His genuine enthusiasm gave me the incentive to take my plan to a patent lawyer. Dad financed it for me and we came home with a patent protection good for six months.

163

The following week, I got a lift over to the field at Astoria and talked to an aeronautics mechanic. He agreed, the plan was good. His job kept him so busy I knew it would be a while before he got the new control finished. I settled down to wait. Months passed. I began to worry about the patent protection running out before the control was done.

One day the mechanic said, "You'll need an airplane to try it out."

A friend in Astoria who was not flying at the time agreed to loan his Piper. It had the kind of stick control we needed.

"I'd better renew the patent protection," I told the mechanic.

"Aw, wait until you see if it works in the air. No use getting a patent until we find out if the thing is worth it."

To our dismay, the next issue of one of the flying magazines came out with a description of the very control I had invented. Someone else had gotten ahead of me!

One day a friend of mine went up in a Silvair to do the loops and tailspins and stunts we'd done so many times before. He flew over his girl friend's house to buzz her and give her a thrill. This time when he dove at the house his plane did not pull out.

Sealy and Norton came over to break the news to me. "He dove right into the yard with her watching. Jesus Christ!"

"Killed?" The look on their faces told me the answer.

I experienced my own brush with death. On a sunny afternoon the instructor got me into the plane we were going to use for my lesson. He taxied to the end of the runway and turned the plane into the wind.

"You forgot to check the magnitos," I reminded him.

"Why bother? This plane has just been used. It's already hot so I'm positive everything's in working order. . . ."

We were about to take off when I said firmly, "Look . . . maybe you don't care but I do. Something inside me tells me you better check those mags. It only takes a minute."

164

"OK then, you win." He clamped on the brakes, revved the engine to 2100 RPM and flipped the right and left mag switch back and forth.

"Satisfied? They check out fine." He put the motor on full throttle, pushed the wheel forward to get the tail up. In a matter of seconds he would ease it back partway and we would be in the air. The wheels were bouncing, we were ready to take off . . . and at that moment the motor died.

The instructor braked and we coasted to a stop. He wiped beads of perspiration from his forehead. "You're trembling, Don . . . I admit that was a close one! Lord, it was close!"

Upon examining the plane we discovered someone had turned off the valve from the wing tank. It was one thing we had neglected to check.

"Makes you believe in Something, doesn't it!" exclaimed the pilot. "You obviously had this feeling something was wrong with the plane."

"Call it a premonition," I told him. "I don't know what it was but it felt as if a force outside of me . . . beyond me . . . was guiding me."

The feeling was more overpowering than I dared let on. I sensed an interrelationship not only between person and person but between man and his environment.

Since childhood, I had been disenchanted with an anthropomorphic God who answered the pleadings of His earthly children. (*Oh God, I ast you and ast you and you didn't hear me . . .*) That idea seemed sheer nonsense. But now I felt certain there must be a greater-than-human life force at work in the world. A nonpersonal cosmic energy radiating power. Had I not been in touch with it?

I was sure I had.

How had it happened spontaneously, without seeking on my part? What did it mean? Could it be more than a fleeting extrasensory perception? Would I find it again? Who was I and why was

I subject to such violent storms of depression coming on the heels of creative surges I was unable to control? I asked these questions and many more.

I had always been a reader. Now I began to direct my reading. I read the works of Freud and Carl Jung and Menninger. I read heavy textbooks on mental health and psychology. I read books written for the laymen on *How to Be a Success* and *How to Beat Depression*, and books on making the most of your talents.

At last the librarian threw up her hands and exclaimed, "Donald, you've borrowed every book on the shelves, haven't you? Have you found what you've been looking for?"

"Some. I'm going to keep looking."

I knew one thing. I wanted to go to college.

The family was ready for a change. Mom had closed her dress shop. Except for summer months business was in a slump. My *Shopping News* had folded because a competitor had started another small weekly paper.

We had another blow too. Dad had a heart attack. Through the years, ever since that long siege with pneumonia in Parker, his health had gradually broken. His year at the shipyard hadn't helped it any . . . that work had been physically much too taxing for him. But, though he'd been sick off and on with flu and bronchitis it was the heart attack that made me realize how his health had failed. I thought about it while he recuperated. In a larger city he might find steady, year round work . . . something that was not too much of a strain.

We'd been in Seaside for seven years. It was time to move back to Portland.

*eleven*

FLOYD and his wife, Toni, were still in Minnesota but Jack and his family had settled in Portland. It was to his home we went while Dad hunted for a house and a new job. After the war, the city police force had tightened up its physical requirements. My brother no longer qualified to be on the force. He had that blind eye and he was too short. The county accepted him though, so now he was a deputy sheriff.

As soon as I got into the city, I called the dean's office at the University of Portland and made an appointment.

What would Fr. Hooyber, the dean of students, say when he met a man with a seventh-grade education who was hell bent on going to college? At the doorway of his office, I hesitated. Then I wheeled inside.

For a long time he talked with me. At last he leaned back in his chair and said, "You are late. The fall term has been in session for a week. But . . . I believe you may be qualified to enter as a freshman. I realize you've had no formal high school training. However," he smiled, "there's schooling and then there's education. They are two different matters. Certainly you are a self-educated man. Would you be willing to take some tests? After that we'll know more."

"When?"

"Today, if it can be arranged."

While I waited, he made a telephone call. I felt nervous. I'd had no opportunity to prepare. I'd never seen a college entrance exam.

His voice splintered my thoughts. "Yes, the room is down the hall on this floor . . . last room to the left at the end of the corridor. You need to be there within the next fifteen minutes."

For eight solid hours I took tests. I took the college entrance exams and an IQ test and many others. I took a Couter preference test. Before I went home that night I was dizzy and very very tired. I didn't have the slightest notion whether I'd scored poorly or well.

A day later, I discovered I'd been accepted as a freshman. I was going to college! The campus was crowded with students going through on the GI bill so I did not feel like an oddity, although I was in my late twenties.

"I'm going to major in music and my minor will be speech and parliamentary procedure," I informed my astounded family. We laughed when we heard how I had come out on the Couter preference test. I'd scored 98% in music, 96% in persuasive arts, 93% in art, 69% in social work, and less than 1/2 of 1% in business aptitude. The test was merely an indication of where my interests lay, but Dad seized the chance to tease me.

"That tells you one thing. You might as well forget about being a big shot in the business world!"

Nothing was farther from my mind than business. I wanted to do something in music. Not the cheap kind of entertainment I'd listened to in taverns and clubs but high quality stuff.

I was not Roman Catholic. I was out of touch with formal religion. But the priests at this Catholic university treated me with

168

warmth and respect. I was given a complete scholarship, no strings attached. Fr. Hooyber jockeyed classes so I could get to them.

"This English class normally meets on the second floor, but we'll just do a bit of room switching, Don, so you can make it without any trouble."

Aware it would take time for me to learn a discipline of study, he suggested I could audit any courses I wanted and earn college credits later. I protested. I wanted to take everything for credit. That was why I was there.

The university provided a chauffeur for my car. I paid not a cent. The boy who took the job had been having difficulty with arthritis so we worked out a perfect arrangement. He had free use of the car as long as he was willing to chauffeur me back and forth to classes and meetings. This was not Cora, the old cut-down Chevvy sedan, but a newer automobile I'd purchased before leaving Seaside.

"Might as well keep it at your house to use for dates or whatever you need it for. I'll call you any time I need to borrow it back."

I struggled to keep up my studies. I found music history and music theory difficult and ended up receiving a flunking grade for the year in both subjects. The history was hard because I had never had the discipline of learning great masses of facts. I discovered, too late, that a large part of music theory had to do with chords. Most of the students in the class had had years of training on a chordal instrument such as piano or organ or both. I had never played a chordal instrument because I could not use both hands. Without this previous knowledge, the theory class was a losing battle.

Music appreciation was a different story though. I had absolute pitch and had no trouble listening to and analyzing various pieces of music.

In speech and parliamentary procedure I was at the head of the class. At midyear, my instructor came to me.

"You know quite a bit about radio, Don. In fact you've had

more actual experience than I've got myself. I was wondering if you'd be interested in helping me start a radio course here at the university. What do you say?''

Of course I said yes. The only problem was the room they picked to convert into a studio. At the time the available space was located on the third floor of Howard Hall. And how would I get up those stairs?

A college buddy, Jerry Hagen, offered to pack me up. He never missed a day that entire spring term. A large and muscular fellow, fresh from the submarine corps, he'd meet me at the bottom step and carry me up the three long flights.

To begin with, we had no real transmitter. The college would supply that later. But we partitioned the large room with glass, making it look like an actual studio. With mikes and public address system, we were able to ''broadcast'' programs to various points on the campus.

During the year I came to grips with one fact. Music theory was over my head. Maybe I could do a great job leading dance bands . . . I was playing my horn in different combos on the weekends. I knew a lot about music, I loved music, but the abstract, technical part was not for me. I was flunking miserably so I changed my major to speech and parliamentary procedure.

Mom had been working in a nursing home. Dad had found a job in a local hardware store. Once again we'd settled in our favorite part of Portland, the St. Johns area, across the river from Vancouver.

Late in the spring, my father had another heart attack. I went in to see Fr. Hooyber.

''I'm going to have to drop out and find a way to support my family for a while. This year at the university has been great for me. . . .''

I felt I might be letting him down after he'd been generous enough to bypass regulations and admit me as a student.

''When your father is better you may want to finish your studies. . . .''

170

I knew in my heart I would not be coming back. Perhaps to take a course here and there, but not to matriculate for a college degree. Dad's health was failing. He would need my help.

I wanted to trade in the car I was using for a different model. I looked over several on a used car lot and selected a 1941 Oldsmobile. A mechanic from the shop across the street noticed my wheelchair. He came over to chat.

"How are you going to drive that?"

"I'll get someone to convert it to hand controls eventually." I had already decided that, even before I knew how I would pay for the damn thing. It was that old sense of determination . . . somehow I'd do it.

"I'll fix it for you."

I was pleased but said, "I don't have a cent to pay you."

"I'm not interested in the money. I'd be happy to do it."

A thrill went through me. At last I'd learn to drive a car!

Jack, when he heard about my new venture, was set against it. "You're a fool, Don. I can promise you one thing. If you do get a license, I'll never ride with you. And what's more, no member of my family will ride with you either. It's too dangerous."

It was Jerry Hagan who taught me how to drive. My car with hand controls gave me a greater degree of mobility than I'd ever known before. By using a small, sturdy board to slide in and out of the seat, I need not depend on any other person to lift me in. I was free to come and go at will! That was a magnificent triumph.

Judge Pezenik flashed into my head . . . old Pezenik coming down the Main Street of Parker with his wheelchair strapped onto the back of his Cadillac . . . my first realization a man in a wheelchair could drive a car. I remembered, too, the car salesman who had taken me out in such a vehicle when I was a teen-ager, and the longing I'd felt at the time . . . and the longing eating at me through the ensuing years when I owned cars that others must drive for me.

This Oldsmobile was different than flying. I loved flying but it was out of reach right now. I had not finished the hours I would need for my pilot's license. What was the use when it would be years before I could afford a plane? But this car with hand controls was real. It was mine.

At last I could go any place I wanted to go!

During the following year, the state rehabilitation office paid for a course I took in executive bookkeeping. I hated that course but grit my teeth and got through it.

"Why do you continue if you hate it so?" wondered Mom one night when I'd been beefing about it.

"Why? I suppose because it isn't a bad skill to have . . . bookkeeping."

I spun from job to job, unable to support myself fully, seeking for something that would pay better. I worked with a roofing contractor, I worked in the Customer Service department at Sears Roebuck, and then I landed a job as disk jockey on a daily, hourlong show at KVAN, a radio station across the river in Vancouver, Washington.

The transmitter for the station was at Smith Lake on our side of the river. It was an easy matter to run a direct line into the studio I set up in our own home. Music and radio . . . once again I would combine the two things I loved best.

In Portland, even more than in Seaside, a disk jockey's life was considered glamorous. I rode through town looking for customers to purchase advertising time on the new Don Kirkendall show. I worked late into the night on commercials and the clever patter I needed to fill gaps between records.

I got the idea of taping conversations with interesting personalities and using them on the show. One of the first persons I interviewed was Jack's boss, the sheriff, Terry Schrunk. He had humor, he was colorful, he was a success, so I taped interviews with other local characters. Gradually I discovered ways to meet celebrities who were nationally known.

172

When I heard the Globe Trotters were in town I went down to the Civic Auditorium to talk to the famous stars who took part in the review at half time.

I made the rounds of supper clubs, especially a place called Amatos, and taped more interviews. I met Guy Lombardo, Patty Page, Eddie Fisher, and a pianist I admired very much, Earl Hines.

Something about a disk jockey appeals to youngsters. Soon kids listening to my midafternoon show began to form fan clubs. One set called themselves the Cadillac Kids. They hounded the station with telephone calls and letters and requests for special recordings. Older people wrote in to ask me to make announcements. New stores invited me to come tape their Grand Openings.

I was building a reputation. It thrilled me to learn I was Number 2 Portland Disk Jockey on the Nielson rating.

Because I was unable to go up and down steps, my advertising clientele was severely limited. Before I could get inside to an elevator I often came face to face with an insurmountable staircase.

I settled for advertisers in stores opening directly onto the street with no steps to navigate. Until Charlie, the owner of a used car lot, thought of a way. A tall, heavyset American Indian, with hair combed straight back off his forehead, Charlie was one of my most amiable clients. He would come out to the car and stand there yakking, any time I stopped by.

"Don, you need a beautiful girl to go up and down the steps and get the customers for you," he joked.

Inside my brain something clicked.

"Charlie, that isn't such a bad idea! I wish I'd thought of it sooner!"

That very afternoon I called a model agency. The girl at the desk took down the information and said briskly:

"I can send one of our models for an interview tomorrow at 10:00 A.M. Would you be free to see her then?"

The following morning, promptly at the appointed hour, the doorbell rang. In came a good-looking female, dressed in the height of fashion. The glossy brown hair under the stovepipe hat hung shoulder length. She was wearing a stylish lightweight paisley coat and high heels. I judged her to be in her late twenties. To my surprise, at her side, clothed with the same impeccable taste, was a little girl.

The model introduced herself. "I am Mary Ann Hand, and this is my daughter, Normandie. We call her Nomie. I was told you are looking for a girl to help you in your business."

I explained the situation. After a few questions she agreed to take the job.

While we got acquainted, Nomie explored around my wheelchair, setting first one small shoe and then the other on the footrests. Finally she ended up where she'd wanted to be in the first place . . . in my lap.

"Nomie! Get down!" her mother chided.

"I don't mind. I've got nephews who like to climb up here too," I assured her.

And so it was with a small golden head snuggled against my shoulder that I ended my first encounter with Mary Ann.

Charlie's idea paid off. Mary Ann added sparkle to my show. She accompanied me everyplace, pushing my wheelchair into areas I could not possibly go without assistance. When we faced a staircase, she handled the appointment with the prospective client alone in a businesslike manner.

She arranged for a sitter to take care of four-year-old Nomie and her six-year-old brother, Greg, in order to be free to attend the interviews I was constantly setting up. Often when I worked late into the night on fresh copy for commercials, she remained at the studio to help.

I wondered how I had managed without her. I called her my Girl Friday.

One person did not appreciate the attractive model I'd hired.

This was my current girl friend, Sally Finey. As disk jockey, my press pass was an open sesame to major night spots. Mary Ann was beginning to usurp Sally's place as my escort.

"Damn it!" I exploded. "This is strictly a business arrangement. She's just gotten a divorce, she's got two kids to think about. Why are you so jealous?"

"Ha!" Sally sniffed and tossed her head in an enigmatic gesture. "If she stays on, you needn't count on me being around any more."

Just the same, she continued to date me, taking ugly digs at Mary Ann whenever possible. Her possessiveness began to cloy.

Mary Ann was an intelligent and beautiful girl. Easy to be with. Fun. We worked well together. So well, as a matter of fact, that she confided she had this special feeling . . . if we kept on working together we could accomplish anything we set out to do.

"Anything!" she repeated with shining eyes.

I knew she was referring to the job. A second marriage was far from her mind. But I knew, too, that she thought I was a hard boss, very masculine . . . those were her words . . . and I was flattered.

She needed time off to look for a house. She wanted to find one close to the job, in order to avoid a long bus ride each evening.

"I'll drive you. I know this neighborhood," I offered.

We hunted a long time. At last we came to a tiny dwelling located in back of a larger one, with a third house still farther back. The sign in the window said "For rent . . . see landlord in house to the rear."

"Those two diamond-shaped windows in front look like eyes," laughed Mary Ann. "It's darling."

"Take it," I advised. "Looks as if it's made for you and the children. It's hardly bigger than a doghouse."

I had noticed immediately that the house had one low front step. If I decided to pay a visit, I could do so with ease.

She hesitated. "Shouldn't I look inside and see what it's like before I rent it?"

"Of course, go ahead."

The back yard was a hayfield, too tall to walk through, so Mary Ann ran around on the sidewalk and knocked on the land-lord's door.

Presently she came again to the car.

"The large house in front is already rented. This one is only thirty-five dollars a month. The landlord and his wife are sweet. Italian. And so friendly! They're coming over with the key."

In a few minutes she had thoroughly inspected the house. She returned to the car ecstatic.

"It's a converted garage, fixed up during the war when hous-ing was so scarce. It's just right for us . . . a bedroom in the loft for the kids, and a foldaway in the living room for me; the dearest little kitchenette, and a shower and toilet—no sink except the one in the kitchen."

She climbed back into the car, chuckling. "I've already named it. Pup House, that's what I'll call it."

Shortly after we found Pup House, we were driving out to the transmitter at Smith Lake one afternoon when I could resist the urge no longer. Catching Mary Ann completely off guard, I slammed on the brakes, pulled her close to me and gave her a good, long kiss.

"Ooooooh! Donald!" she gasped. "I've never been kissed like that in my whole life!" Her eyes glistened as she said it. Two pink spots of color had appeared in her high cheekbones.

"I'm going to marry you some day," I announced as matter of factly as I could.

"That's sweet of you to say that," she murmured. "But Don, I don't have marriage in mind."

Whenever we attended evening functions, I drove her home. One night the motor of the Oldsmobile died as I pulled up in front of Pup House. I sighed.

"How in the name of God will I find someone to come out and fix it at this hour of the night?"

"You can use my telephone. Come in and have some coffee while you hunt for a garage that's open."

She hurried to the back of the car and got my folding chair. Then she waited while I twisted and shoved onto the slide board and from there into the chair. Inside the house, she made coffee in her wee kitchen. It was actually little more than a corner of the living room with a partition to provide extra wall space.

Pup House was quiet. The children must be sound asleep upstairs in the loft. But as I made my phone calls, I began to hear giggles and whispers. Once I caught a glimpse of two towheads peeping at me from the stairs. In a flash they disappeared. Five minutes later they were back, convulsed with giggles.

I heard Mary Ann attempting to sound stern.

"Children! Go back to bed!"

"Greg, Normandie! did you hear what I said? Go back to . . . oh well, you might as well come down here and say 'hello' to my boss before you go upstairs again."

"A man'll be over from the Ace Garage within half an hour," I reported after much phoning.

This time I had two children instead of one in my wheelchair with me. Greg was openly impressed.

"Why do you have to use it?" he demanded. "Can I try it? Show me how it works . . . oh, that's neat!"

Before I went home that night, I knew I'd been accepted as a hero.

Mom and Dad had been observing our growing relationship. Diffident toward them in the beginning, soon Mary Ann had come to have warm feelings. Once she admitted her first impression to me and we laughed.

"The first time I ever saw your father, I thought he was the meanest man I'd ever seen! And . . . and . . . I had your mother pegged as . . . sort of a social clubwoman type. But now. . .''

"Now?"

"I love them."

"And how about me?" I was busy wooing her with a blues trumpet.

She pirouetted around the room . . . she had been a dancer since childhood and was very graceful . . . "I'm fond of you, Don. I guess I'm in love with you. Being with you is like going to a foreign country."

"Why?" I asked curiously.

One foot in midair, she paused, then came over and sat down beside me. "I was brought up in such a ladylike way—conservative—everything had to be just so. I've never met anyone as natural as you. Or as real. You do what you feel is right inside, not what society dictates."

"Everything just so." I smiled. "You mean like whole milk in your coffee instead of canned?"

A few months ago, Mary Ann had been shocked to discover our Kirkendall family had never used anything but canned milk in our coffee.

"That was fine back on the farm when you were poor," she'd told me privately. "But it isn't necessary anymore. Why don't you get them to try whole milk, Don?"

I ended up being the one to take her suggestion. Now I was a staunch advocate of whole milk in coffee. But an odd thing had happened. Guilty about being critical, Mary Ann had tried canned milk in *her* coffee one day and from that time on would drink nothing else.

She blushed. "Play me some more blues."

"Wish granted. But first *you* do another dance for *me*. . . ."

"If we do get married," she commented on another day, "I'm glad we can live with your parents. That way they'll be able to help me over the rough spots, getting used to the way you manage the wheelchair and bath. . . ."

178

"Hell, Mary Ann!" I exploded. "I promised myself if I ever married again I wouldn't live in my parents' house. No way! This time I'll have a home of my own and some privacy."

Neither of us wanted a big wedding. We talked about sneaking away without letting a single person know, not even members of the Kirkendall clan. In the end we had to tell Mom and Dad because a one-hour-a-day disk jockey, famous though he may be, earns little. I was broke. I borrowed the money for our wedding-license from my father.

"There wasn't enough left over to buy you a wedding ring," I told Mary Ann sadly.

"Oh pooh! I don't care! *We* know we're married, don't we?"

Long had I looked forward to our wedding night. Mary Ann's background was Victorian enough that, although both of us had been married and divorced, we had done nothing more than a little parking and smootching. But, after the wedding a strange and rather amusing thing happened. Weariness overtook us, combined with a deep sense of belonging to one another at last. We snuggled together in the big bed in the living-room of Pup House and fell into a dreamless and refreshing sleep, leaving our first real love-making until morning.

My move into Pup House spurred the children into a wild and enthusiastic mood. Excitement mounted during the next two days. They yelled, they quarreled. In a matter of hours they'd changed from two well-behaved kids into monsters. They banged my wheelchair, they fought to be the first in my lap, they bawled when it came time for bed, they tested my patience in every conceivable way.

At the end of the second day, I roared, "For the love of Mike, Mary Ann, what has happened? Why don't you *do* something?"

I was seething. Couldn't she see how disruptive they had become?

"*You* do it, Don," she said in a quiet voice. "You're the father in this household now."

I was taken aback. I had not fully realized the implications of being a parent.

"All right," I agreed. "But if I do it, it's going to be in my own way, understand? No interference from the sidelines."

The next time Greg got sassy, I leaned out of my wheelchair and with my good left arm swept him up and turned him across my knee.

"Na . . . na, na . . . na, na . . .na!" Nomie danced in front of me, giggling as her brother stumbled sobbing up the stairs. In a flash she received the same treatment amid howls of anguish.

"Now then, young lady, go finish your crying in bed. And don't come down until you can behave yourself," I growled.

I heaved a sigh and wiped the perspiration from my forehead. "They'll probably keep a mile away from me now," I said to Mary Ann.

To my surprise it wasn't ten minutes before the two of them trotted down the stairs and gave me a forgiving kiss on the forehead.

"Two's plenty! Thank God we don't have to worry about having a large family!"

Long ago in a doctor's office I'd been told I was sterile and would never father a child. At the time I hadn't felt too upset about this. I'd already proved to myself I could have a normal sexual relationship anyway.

"How strange," murmured Mary Ann a month later.

"What's strange?"

"If you hadn't told me we couldn't have children, I'd swear I was pregnant. I sure have that special feeling. . . . "

"Impossible," I said laughing. Then I added, alarmed, "If something's wrong, you go in for a checkup, hear?"

"Heck, I'm not sick." She laughed. "It's just a funny feeling."

We found it difficult to mix our disk jockey and Girl Friday roles with marriage. The demands were too numerous.

"Any early appointments tomorrow, boss?" Mary Ann let out a sigh of contentment when I shook my head "no."

"Then let's sleep in and have waffles and coffee in bed. There's plenty of room for the children to crawl in at the other end."

At that point the phone would ring.

"It's KVAN . . . they want us to meet Eddie Fisher's plane and have a breakfast interview. Tomorrow morning at seven."

"Nuts!"

At times we were in our bathrobes, reading aloud to each other in bed when it rang. "Tape and interview with Earl Hines. In an hour? Sure thing . . ."

Wash . . . shave . . . clean clothes . . . hide your fatigue under a facade of pep . . . drop two sleeping children off at Grandma's . . . by the time we get to Amatos both of us will be looking livelier . . . come on, old girl, we'll be back in bed by two. . . ."

We had to admit, the glamour had gone out of it.

"I'd feel different," I muttered one night, "if I was rolling in dough." But it wasn't that way.

One thing saved me after an hour of small talk with the glittering stars, and that was the other kind of interview, sometimes funny, often serious, with local civic leaders. With the latter I did not have to "put on the dog." I could relax. In the end, they turned out to be every bit as interesting as the more famous people.

Take an old friend . . . the sheriff, Terry Schrunk, who accepted an occasional invitation to be on the show. Those times the repartee was quick, unforced, funny.

Once we began our hour on an unusual note of hilarity. Terry strode into the studio as we were about to go on the air and clapped a pair of real handcuffs on my Girl Friday.

Mary Ann's surprised laughter could be heard all over Portland as listeners tuned in.

"I'm going to take you into custody as soon as you're finished here at the studio." The sheriff tried hard to sound gruff.

"Tell me why."

"It has been called to my attention you are a horse thief. The technician at the transmitter says he caught you redhanded. On a stolen horse." (More laughter.)

Mary Ann interrupted to explain to her listening audience: "When the boss and I drove out to get the records today, there was this beautiful dappled gray horse in the field, and nobody in sight. Well, gang, I grew up with horses and this was one creature I simply couldn't resist. . . ."

"Before I could say a word," I interjected, "Girl Friday was out of the car and riding off bareback. But sheriff, it was a borrowed horse, not a stolen one."

It was pure corn but our fans loved every minute of it.

We'd been married a little over two months. Mary Ann said for the second time, "Don . . . there's no way to prove it yet, but I do feel pregnant."

"Too pregnant to go to a talent show?" I teased. I knew what she was saying couldn't be true. "The president's Commission on the Handicapped is in town. They want to put on a benefit a week from Saturday down at one of the big hotels." I smirked. "Because I'm a well-known disk jockey, I've been asked to MC."

"I thought you refused to be classified as a handicapped person."

"Right. But I accepted this on the basis of being talented, rather than being handicapped. I'll take my trumpet along."

A lady named Mrs. Fitzrandolph-Williams had charge of the evening. She was so overly exuberant, so sickeningly sweet, we dubbed her simply "Mrs. Fits."

A few days before the event was to take place, we met with her to discuss the entertainment.

"What should I wear?" I asked.

"Dahling," she gushed, looking me over as though I was someone to be pitied, "just dress as well as you can."

I arrived at the affair in a rented tux. Mary Ann looked stunning in a strapless ice-blue brocaded evening gown. Mrs. Fits saw us at the edge of the crowd. She swept over and shook a finger at us, coyly, murmuring, "Oh, you're soooooo *pretty!*"

It was a gala evening. Or it would have been, without Mrs. Fits. During the dinner she spotted our table and came and leaned over my shoulder to whisper in my ear:

"I understand your wife is a marvelous dancer. Do you suppose she'd do us the honor to perform during the evening?"

"I don't believe she'd want to do that," I whispered back. "At any rate, not right now."

The program ran smoothly. I came on at the end to close with a trumpet solo . . . "September Song." I had not played professionally for many months. But somehow I got into the spirit of the evening and gave it my best. When I played the last note I heard a moment of silence, then thunderous applause. People gathered around to rave over my solo and to tell me what a fine job I'd done as master of ceremonies.

In the background, Mrs. Fits' voice called from the stage . . .

"Yoo hoo . . . Donald . . . May I tell?"

Tell what? I didn't know. I was busy with people asking questions. "Sure, go ahead." Totally unaware of what she had in mind.

She clapped her hands to get everyone's attention.

"It is my pleasure to announce this evening that our *Beyootiful* Mrs. Kirkendall cannot dance tonight because she is expecting a baby."

I saw Mary Ann blush. She scrunched down in her seat to avoid stares, slipping so low that she ended up under the table, a crumpled heap of blue brocade.

"We're not sure about it ourselves," we told Mrs. Fits as we bid her good bye a few minutes later. "It's too early to tell. Much too early." ("How did she know?" I whispered to Mary Ann . . . "I didn't tell her . . .")

"Oh dearie, don't worry about it. My little girl was an eight months' baby." She winked.

183

Mary Ann drowned her out. She said stiffly and loud enough for everyone to hear: "Ours will be full term. We were married last April and, if I am pregnant, the baby will not arrive until January." Without another word she pushed my wheelchair out the door.

"That woman!" she muttered on the way home. "That woman!"

I took her to the finest obstetrician in the city. We sat in his posh office waiting for our turn and looking at the women in dressy maternity clothes. The receptionist beckoned us into a corner.

As kindly as she could, in a low voice, she broke the news to us. She could see we'd have a hard time paying this doctor's bills. He charged a high sum to deliver a baby. She gave us the name of a hospital, St. Vincent's, and a doctor who would be far less expensive.

We left the clinic at St. Vincent's after our first appointment, knowing Mary Ann was indeed pregnant, and assured our baby would be born on Catholic charity. On the way home Mary Ann breathed a thankful sigh.

"You didn't graduate from the university. And neither of us has been confirmed in the Roman Catholic faith. Yet they're so kind to us . . . I don't understand."

"I do," I answered. "If a person has a real need, it doesn't make any difference to the priest if he is Catholic or heathen. My year at the university was one of the best in my life. And look at the way they've treated my father!" Like Mary Ann, I felt a deep sense of gratitude.

The university had provided a part-time job for Dad Kirkendall, first as a dishwasher, then as a night watchman. The dean and the president watched him make his rounds. They saw how feeble he was becoming. They heard reports he was shuffling badly. Sometimes he fell. Instead of firing him, they found another way to handle the matter.

Late one afternoon, Dad dropped by Pup House for a cup of coffee with Mary Ann on his way to work.

"Son of a bitch. Those college students treat me like I was the Pope. Why, every time I stumble, a couple of them come running over to pick me up."

Mary Ann looked sideways at him. She told me about it later when I came in.

"I asked if he wasn't lonely, late at night. I've been worrying over those spills he takes. But," she smiled, "he says someone is always on hand to help him if he needs it. Don, do you suppose the dean has actually assigned students to follow him and see that nothing happens?"

"No way of proving it. But I wouldn't put it past him."

We knew we were going to need more money. In October, the Don Kirkendall show went off the air. I took a part-time job with an insurance company. In a fit of depression, I said to Mary Ann, "Gosh darn it, I wish for once I could find something with a salary that would support us. This is terrible!"

For a moment she was silent. Then slowly, she turned and looked me in the eye. "Don, the trouble with you is this: you don't know how to work!"

*twelve*

---

" "W HO are you kidding?" I yelled in fury.

Abruptly, I left the house. Up and down the streets of the St. John's area I rolled, boiling mad. The nerve of her! Saying a thing like that!

But I knew she had spoken the truth. I had never worked at a full-time job, earning enough of a salary to support myself and a wife and children. Never! And I was in my thirties now, a grown man. The thought appalled me.

I wheeled back home and got into the car. I'd show her I could do it. I'd show her!

This time I ended up with not one but two jobs in different offices. During the day I did desk work and answered the telephone at a U Rent auto place. At night I made appointments, by phone, for an insurance firm. I was out of bed at 6:00 a.m. I worked fourteen hours a day and paid every one of our bills.

"There!" I announced with satisfaction on a Saturday morning. I let Nomie and Greg have the honor of stamping the envelopes and mailing them. "The next problem is where will we put the baby in a house this size?"

Mary Ann smiled. "I've figured it out." She went over to the little piano and tugged it out from the wall. "See Don, this nook behind the piano will be big enough to fit a crib."

With the bills paid, there was money left over to buy Christmas presents. I had bought something special for my wife. Christmas morning she looked with curiosity at the large box with her name on it under the tree. She laughed as she discovered a smaller box inside and one still smaller inside of that. When she reached the last very small box, her cheeks grew pink. "Oh Donald! I know what it must be . . . yes! Yes! A wedding band!"

The day spilled over with warmth and laughter. We would be going over to Dad and Mom Kirkendall's for dinner. But there was time first to relax at Pup House, time for the children to enjoy their toys. Greg zoomed around with his new dump truck. But small Nomie brought her doll and settled down by my chair. A motherly child, she loved to take care of me. Today she busied herself lifting my legs, one at a time, and slipping my shoes off and putting my Christmas slippers on and off my feet.

"Oh Daddy!" she squealed after a while. "Isn't this fun?"

"Yes indeed. And know what?" I glanced over at Mary Ann. "Your new baby sister or brother will be arriving in less than a month."

That night when Mary Ann stretched out on the bed I rested my hand lightly on her swollen belly to feel the baby kick.

"Active little devil, isn't he!"

"Are you glad that doctor was wrong when he said you'd be sterile?"

"Hell, nobody can fool a doctor like I can, Mary Ann. Did I ever tell you about the time I thought I had appendicitis? One look at my X ray and they said, 'Kirkendall, your insides are so twisted around that we can't find anything. Jeez, man, there's no way to tell if you even have an appendix!' One doctor poked me here and there and said, 'If you say it hurts, it hurts!' Medical people gave up on me long ago!''

In January the weather turned cold and blustery and we were surprised by snow. Many winters Portland does not see snow. But this time it was a doozy of a storm.

I began to get itchy about driving Mary Ann to the hospital. How would I get out of the car to help her? Unless a miracle happened and it cleared before her time came.

"I'll ask Mom and Dad to stand by. They can go up with us."

"Please, Don. This is our private affair. I don't want another person but you."

I stared at her dumbfounded. Apparently it hadn't occurred to her that it would be difficult, impossible maybe, for me to maneuver the car on an icy hill.

But she seemed certain it would pose no problem. Since she felt that way, I decided not to say a word.

We made it to the hospital. Mary Ann gave birth to a baby girl. We named her Kip Suzanne. I went home, exultant, to tell the family. Three days later, I received a telephone call at work.

"Kip and I are ready for you to come get us," announced Mary Ann. "Tell your boss you'll have to take the rest of the afternoon off. Oh, and Don, please don't bring anyone else along. I want it to be just you."

Inwardly, I groaned. The road up to St. Vincent's Hospital would be icier than ever. Both snow and rain had fallen since she'd entered the maternity wing.

I made it up the hill, into the parking lot. My folding wheelchair was in the seat beside me. I set it outside the door and, using the sliding board, wormed safely into it. I'd never be able to maneuver myself over the ice and ridges of snow to the hospital doorway without some help though.

As soon as a man came out, his overcoat collar turned up

188

against the wind, I hollered unabashedly, "Hey, Mister, would you mind lending a hand with my chair?"

Inside, I rolled down the hall to Mary Ann's room. "I've got you signed out. Everything's taken care of. We can go." She never guessed what an undertaking it had been.

"That's fine." It was as if I conquered ice and drifts of snow in a wheelchair every day of my life. "Look, Donald, isn't she a queen?" She held out our baby so I could take a peep.

A nurse accompanied us out to the car and took me and the chair skillfully across the snow.

Going down the icy hill was much more difficult than the journey up it had been. I went slow, but the car skidded anyhow. If only we didn't get stuck! From hidden depths, I muttered a spontaneous prayer: "If Somebody *is* out there, please get us off this hill!"

Next to me, Mary Ann cuddled our infant daughter and smiled a complacent smile. Convinced I'd make it. When we rolled off the hill onto the highway, I sucked in a deep breath. The road was a sheet of ice but not as treacherous as the hill. The baby started to whimper. Mary Ann unbuttoned her blouse and began to nurse.

My turn to smile!

Greg and Nomie inspected their new sister from top to bottom, admiring the tiny toes and perfectly formed ears and wispy hair and shell-like fingernails. Mom clucked like an old hen and Dad offered the baby a horny knuckle, which she naturally refused.

"Jeerusalem!" He hitched up his pants. "She's really something!"

Mary Ann held her close, offering her milky nipple at the first cry of distress, and wiping her little ass at least two dozen times a day. But no member of the Kirkendall family knew a greater joy than mine.

Carefully, I balanced my daughter in my lap. Each time I

189

wheeled by the piano, I listened to the coos and gurgles issuing from the crib behind it.

"Just think!" I bragged at the supper table. "In less than a year I've become the father of three very beautiful children. Now that takes talent, doesn't it?"

"Either talent or a scandal," commented Mary Ann.

The rest of the family grinned. Nomie cast me an adoring look and bustled away to find my slippers.

Spring in Pup House was a mellow season. The heavy rains ceased. Saturated with moisture, the yard turned fresh and green. The cherry tree bloomed and the air had a fragrant smell.

The entire neighborhood congregated in our yard to play. Out in back was a broken-down old shack the children had named Horse House because of the horse shoe tacked over the door. Horse House provided a haven for many of those mysterious games of childhood grown-ups know nothing about. Early in the summer we bought a pool eight feet in diameter and here the children and I spent many a Saturday afternoon splashing and rough housing and playing games.

We'd turned in our old car. Now we owned a station wagon, complete with the necessary hand controls. In addition, we bought a tent. On weekends we camped in parks from one end of Oregon to the other, and up into the state of Washington.

Jack's boss, Terry Schrunk, was running for mayor this year. Early in the fall, we offered to help him campaign. We put plenty of extra miles on the station wagon, delivering pamphlets and bumper stickers.

"He won!" shouted Mary Ann on election day. "He won!"

"He'll make a hell of a good mayor," I told her. We both chuckled, recalling some of the good times we'd had with Terry during my disk jockey days. Especially the afternoon he'd handcuffed my Girl Friday.

My old wheelchair, Josephine, had finally given up the ghost.

As soon as Kip could crawl, she had learned to climb on Josephine when I was using my folding chair. By the hour she teetered and rocked contentedly. Now the ancient wheelchair was so wobbly it was of little use to me.

"I'll order an electric wheelchair this time Mary Ann. They're expensive but I can put a down payment on it and pay the rest on time."

I selected a large, heavy wheelchair. It ran on batteries. When the batteries were removed, it could be folded and set in the car. The back had a zipper, making it possible for me to slide out onto the portable toilet we'd purchased for camping trips. This adjustable back would come in handy, too, when I visited in homes or motels and found myself with a bed that was difficult to get into any other way. The chair was a sturdy one, built for rough terrain. Mary Ann smiled when she saw the hard rubber tires.

"Thank goodness! No more stinky tires!" She was referring to the tires on Josephine. In my poorer days I had sealed the punctures in those tires with canned milk. This made a good sealer but whenever I had a blowout—what an odor!

"It's $850, a lot of money. But, unlike cars, wheelchairs have no built in obsolescence. They're made to last."

There was something big and strong and masculine about that chair, so I named it Herman.

Like the first car with hand controls, my new electric wheelchair was a milestone. I could go much farther without getting fatigued. I no longer had to depend on someone being around to boost me over rough spots. With a slight push on the hand lever, I could go forward, backward, right or left, fast or slow.

The children were intrigued. They begged for rides. They thought Herman was marvelous. But, strangely, Mary Ann did not. Sensing an undercurrent of resentment, I asked her what was wrong.

"Oh Don!" Her eyes misted. "You'll think I'm an idiot

191

. . . but I need you so. And . . . and now that you have that chair, you'll be so darn independent you won't be needing me half as much as you used to.''

"Come here, woman!" I grabbed her and yanked her into my lap and gave her a long smooch. "There are a few things an electric wheelchair *can't* do. I still need you very much, understand?''

To take the place of the two jobs I'd had, I found one that paid as much and I accepted it. This time the wages were decent but the working conditions left much to be desired. I would be a Food Counselor in a Frozen Food Locker on the other side of town. My "office" was a tiny room on the second floor of the building. In order for me to get up there, someone must lift me out of my folding wheelchair and place me on a kitchen chair in the meat lift. No room to fit even a frozen slab of beef beside me. Another worker would fold my chair and deliver it later when I was settled in my office for the day. My cubbyhole had no windows, no ventilation, and, once I was up there, I must spend the entire day. No coffee break, no way to go to the bathroom. I kept three or four empty milk cartons on hand for this purpose. At the end of the day, someone would empty them for me.

"It's terrible!" exclaimed Mary Ann. "Suppose the building catches on fire? There's no way to get you out.''

"That's right. But of course it's not going to catch on fire,'' I reassured her. Inside, I, too, dreaded the idea of spending my days in that awful cubbyhole.

My job was tedious. It was my task to telephone the entire list of customers each month and coax them into purchasing sides of beef, steaks, turkeys, frozen vegetables.

One good thing . . . I was making enough money to pay our bills. I felt happy about that.

Kip was not yet two when Mary Ann announced she was pregnant again.

"This time try for a boy," urged Greg. "I'd like a brother. We got enough girls.''

192

"I'll do my best," Mary Ann promised, mussing his hair. "But in the end, we'll have to take whatever comes."

Greg's wish came true. The baby was a boy and we named him Kelly. With Kelly we knew only pain. The doctor informed us the first day that he would not live more than a few months. He had been born with a malady that prevented him from digesting food normally. He remained at the hospital long after Mary Ann came home. Later we tried to take care of him ourselves. He wailed constantly and needed around-the-clock care. We grew exhausted.

"The rest of our family needs us too," wept Mary Ann one day. "There must be a better way."

Drained of emotion and energy, we took him to Waverly Baby Home. We knew our baby would not live much longer.

The day Kelly died my boss came up in the meat lift to give me the message.

"You'd better go home, Donald," he said. "Mary Ann will be needing you."

I grieved not for my son Kelly, but for Mary Ann who had borne him inside herself for nine months, had given him passage out of darkness into this world of light, had looked forward to a new baby to cherish, had turned our tiny Pup House upside down preparing for him.

The crib sat empty behind the piano. We folded it and stored it away, shoving the piano back against the wall. Kip had been moved up to share the loft with Nomie, and while waiting for Kelly's arrival, Mary Ann had transformed the large closet near the utility room into a bedroom for Greg.

His own private room! He loved it. Because it was windowless, Mary Ann had hung a curtain in place of the door. She had painted the walls a gaudy yellow. In a surplus store, she found an army cot. After this was set up in the closet room, there was no space for furniture. Greg could reach out of bed to the original closet shelves along the wall and pick whatever toy he wanted without budging.

"A real army cot! Oh boy!" He gloated because nobody else in the neighborhood had a room like his.

"Why does he think a little bitty space like that is so special?" I asked. We were lying awake, talking, in our own living room bed.

"Don't you remember how kids love cubbyholes?" Mary Ann inquired. "They're mysterious . . . but safe. Like a nest. You can cuddle up in them and the giants outside can't reach you."

I thought of the ward at the hospital with its rows of boys. ("Hey Donald, pass the dump truck down and we'll fill it up with cheese . . . Nurse, I need a bed pan . . . hurry, nurse, I can't wait any longer . . . Doctor, what are you going to do, cut me . . . no, no cutting . . .") "I guess I missed the cubbyhole experience," I remarked outloud.

Perhaps I hadn't. I remembered, too, those interior flights into an imaginary world during the long and dreary hospital days. In the end, I too had found a place of my own where nobody else could come.

There is a deep, unreachable grief one must face alone. Exhausted by the emotional turmoil of the past months and the abominable working conditions at the Food Locker, I sank into periods of depression. Neither Mary Ann's dancing . . . in her sadness she still danced . . . nor Nomie's small, firm hands lifting my feet in and out of my slippers brought me out of it.

"The Locker provides no way for growth or change," I pointed out to Mary Ann. "I'm not going anywhere, that's the trouble. I'm stuck. Music as a career is out for me . . . I accepted that after trying it as a major at the university. And radio doesn't seem to be the way I'll make a living. Especially now that television is in. But I sure don't want to stay on as Food Counselor to people buying frozen beef for the rest of my life."

We were sitting in a state park a few miles from the city, watching the children play.

"I've been thinking, Don." Mary Ann leaned down to Kip

who had toddled over, and wiped the baby's runny nose with a crumpled paper napkin. "All of your life you've loved to draw. Why don't you let me work and support the family and you go to art school? You might wind up in commercial art or in teaching, or in some related field. Anyway, it would get you out of this rut."

I mulled over the idea. The more I thought about it, the more I liked it. In a few days we drove downtown to the Portland Museum Art School and talked to the dean. A new term would begin within the next two weeks.

Suddenly Pup House became a hive of activity and planning. I left the Food Locker and found myself a part-time job making appointments by telephone for a building contractor. Mary Ann whisked in and out, checking the children, before continuing with her job search. Grandma Kirkendall calmly pitched in.

"No need to hire a sitter," she advised us. "The two older children will be in school and you can drop Kip at my house each morning."

Thrilled, I went down to the school and registered for classes. Just to cut free of that windowless cubbyhole made me elated. I squandered part of my last paycheck on the special drawing pencils I would need, sticks of charcoal, oil paints, turpentine, linseed oil, pads of drawing paper, a few canvases, and colors. When it came to selecting the oil colors, I could hardly keep from going wild. The very names made me itch to get started . . . cadmium yellow, ultramarine, burnt sienna, raw umber, cobalt blue . . .

Mary Ann came out to the car to help carry the supplies inside. When she saw my purchases, she laughed for joy.

She had news for me. "A very good job . . . I'm going to be a Meter Maid. It's a decent salary and I think I'll like it."

At the Museum Art School I met a host of interesting people: controversial artists like Louis Bunce, one of my teachers who had made a name for himself with his abstract impressionistic mural in the waiting room of the airport; talented students who took their courses seriously; and many others, old and young, male and female, who would always be dabblers. I learned to look at people and inanimate objects in a new way. A crumpled piece of foil separated itself into fascinating planes when I attempted to draw it. I began to notice details I had never seen before . . . the lights and shadows on a wall, the roundness of an orange, the rough texture of its peel, the shadow it cast when it sat, polished by sunlight, on the table. I tried to draw the essence of an orange . . . an apple, green melting into red . . . a basket of eggs.

I saw new details when I looked at people's faces and hands. I studied the way the flesh stretched over the cheekbone, the cleft in the chin, the lines in the forehead and at the corners of the eye. I watched the way various people sat, slumped or erect, weary or ready to move into action at the slightest provocation. I watched Mary Ann in the shower as I had so often watched her before. But this time I saw with a fresh vision . . . the droplets of water running down her neck and shoulders, the twist of her body as she reached to scrub her back with a soapy cloth. I looked with longing at her lithe body dancing nude into the living room and wondered, could I ever learn to catch that subtle beauty with brushes and tubes of color on a canvas?

I looked at my left hand and said to it, "Polio made you what you are. The polio that destroyed the muscle in my right hand brought you into power."

Meter-maiding was a physically exhausting job. Mary Ann grew pale and weary. She had to be on her feet for hours at a time, and out in every kind of weather.

"I walked ten miles today in the rain," she sighed one night. And then she smiled. "Don, it's worth it for you to get to do your art. How much do the models get paid?"

"They get two dollars an hour for modeling nude. One dollar an hour for doing it in clothes."

I read her mind and added quickly, "You can do it in your clothes if you want. They need somebody for Saturday mornings."

She chuckled. "Thanks, boss. That day you can stay home

196

and tend to the children. It'll be a good outing for me and bring in a bit of extra cash. Might even be enough to cover your art supplies."

And so each Saturday morning, she went down to the Museum Art School to model for a drawing class. In clothes. At home she modeled nude for me.

I drew her high cheekbones and angular chin. I drew her auburn hair, sometimes tied back into a single braid with a colored ribbon woven through it, sometimes loose and shining on her bare shoulders. I discovered ways to indicate with charcoal or pencil the graceful lines of her breasts and slender body, those long legs so full of dancing.

One Saturday Mary Ann asked the instructor if she might bring Eo, our dalmation, for the sake of variety. The entire class was delighted, especially when my wife prodded the instructor into paying our dog two dollars an hour because he modeled without a stitch on.

Eventually I let go of my part-time jobs. I wanted to devote more hours to art. I used the children as models whenever I could coax them into sitting still. At times I cajoled them with extra stories of the Black Knight, an endless mystery I invented as I told it and usually saved for a bedtime treat.

I tried self-portraits, staring into the mirror. I did a charcoal bust of Homer, capturing his heavy head of hair, his sensitive face, his unseeing eyes.

I grew to love the familiar smell of linseed oil and turpentine. Blobs of rich color glistened on my palette, waiting to be used. I knew an inexpressible joy each time I streaked enough color on my canvas at last to have the beginning of a picture.

I found I was able to get into a painting and stay there. Inner parts of me emerged, parts I'd never known before. One day a special oil painting was born from this unknown depth. It was a picture of Mother Earth.

We wanted a picture to hang between the two diamond windows. With this in mind, I painted Mother Earth on a horizontal piece of cardboard. The abstract, impressionistic manner seemed an appropriate way to express the surge of feelings and ideas pouring out of me.

Gradually the voluptuous, sleeping figure took shape. I was attempting to show the volcanic forming of the earth during its initial period of gestation. I caught the feeling of rest, too—rest after violence—in my figure of Mother Earth.

I painted her sleeping peacefully as the plants around her began to grow. But the colors themselves were volcanic. For the heavy figure I used a mixture of gray and ochre and blue, with white highlights. I painted the background a fiery cadmium red. A single branch cut across it.

Mary Ann was touched by this painting. She said little but she gazed at it many times, after we'd hung it on the wall between the windows. It was as if a wordless communication took place between person and picture.

Months later, I painted another picture which became well known in our community. Friends visiting in our home either liked it or hated it. The ones who hated it seemed to remain glued to it, fascinated in spite of their aversion. I tried to analyze why it was a controversial picture. Perhaps it was the starkness, the black background, the intense, almost wild look in the subject's eyes. The picture was a portrait of a monk. We had met him quite by accident, this way:

It was winter. Bad weather had kept the family boxed inside our little Pup House.

"Come . . . come . . ." murmured Mary Ann on a Saturday afternoon. "A drive in the country will be just the thing to pep us up."

We left the city behind us and took a road we'd never traveled before. The winter rain had stopped but the day was cold and raw, without sun. For an hour we drove without saying much. The road wound up and down hill over the bleak landscape until we came to a long low building. It looked somewhat like an army barracks.

198

"It has a cross on it," Mary Ann noticed. "It must have some connection with a church. Is it a school? I don't see any sign of life."

"There's cattle over there." I pointed. "And the sign above the door says Our Lady of Guadeloupe. Must be a monastery."

"Yes indeed," said the soft-spoken monk who opened the door when we knocked. "This is a Roman Catholic monastery. I am Brother Matthew, the only one delegated to speak. The rest keep strict silence. However one of us must greet the public."

His nose was red with the cold. The building had no heat. He showed Mary Ann and the children around while I remained in the chapel. There were too many steps for me to explore the rest of the place.

"Some of the brothers do bookbinding," he explained before we left. "Others make furniture."

"What purpose do you have for existing as a monastic order?" inquired Mary Ann.

A distant look came into his eyes. As if he was seeing a vision we could not see. "Our purpose?" he asked gently. "We exist to pray for the rest of the world."

At home I painted a side view portrait of Brother Matthew as I remembered him. I painted him in a flowing white robe, using shades of black and gray, except for the color of his flesh. When I was done, Mary Ann studied it.

"You've managed to get the starkness of that atmosphere. The fierce light in his eye . . . the vision."

Besides life drawing and oil painting, I took a course in commercial art. I had studied at the Museum Art School for nearly a year and a half. I was doing fine in my studies. But, day by day, I could not help noticing Mary Ann's increasing fatigue. She was physically spent from the demands of her job. Along with meter-maiding and modeling, she'd earned extra cash by selling a couple of articles to the newspaper. I had done the ink sketches for the one on her job.

"I don't want any argument about this," I announced one day. "I've told the dean of the art school I have to quit. I'm going back to work, Mary Ann. I can't stand seeing you so tired and half sick."

She looked around at the pictures hanging on the walls of Pup House, the tubes of color, the brushes and sketch pads strewn over my desk. Stricken, she turned to me.

"Oh Don, no!"

"Oh Mary Ann, yes! I want to be the one who is supporting the family. That's my job!"

I tickled her in the ribs and kissed her eyelids until she gave up complaining about my decision. "It won't be so bad, Mary Ann. It's about time the kids had you home for a while. And about time we caught up on our love-making. We've been too busy . . ."

"You don't have to give up painting. You can continue on your own." She brightened at the thought.

"That's the spirit. Be sure you go into the office and give your boss notice tomorrow."

*thirteen*

B Y sheer luck I landed a job as assistant to the credit manager in Anktons Power Plant. The Power Plant sold new furnaces and serviced old ones. It also sold heating oil. It was my job to set up appointments with prospective customers. By telephone, I sold oil and explained anything they wanted to know about new furnaces.

Anktons was a comfortable place to work, except for the bathroom. This was a good distance from the office. My heavy electric wheelchair, Herman, was too big and bulky to fold and transport over there daily. My lightweight folding chair, the one I brought to the office, did not have a crank. I must steer it by pushing the wheel manually. By the time I traversed the length of the power plant to the bathroom and back again to my office, my hand had picked up plenty of dirt from the wheel. I had no way to wash before tackling the paperwork on my desk.

Once again old Pezenik flashed into my mind.

"That guy had a whole wardrobe of wheelchairs," I told Mary Ann. "He left one at the office and one at home, and another at his in-law's house."

Her eyes twinkled. "You're making a good salary, Don, so go ahead and order an extra chair for the office."

My new chair was smaller than Herman but it was another battery operated chair. Again, it was expensive . . . eight hundred dollars. It could be taken apart for trips. Although it did not have the zippered back, it had another feature that would prove valuable in many situations . . . removable arms. Because it was light, it would not go over rough terrain like my heavy chair. Nor could somebody boost me up and down steps in it. The arms of the chair were likely to lift off unexpectedly in the process. But, as a chair to leave at the office, it was perfect.

For the first few days, Mary Ann looked as if she was waiting for something to happen. Finally she gave me a peculiar look. "You haven't named it yet."

I laughed. "Didn't think about it. This one is just a utilitarian chair . . . I don't seem to feel any need to name it. Maybe Herman'll be the last of my chairs to have that distinction."


During the first months at Anktons I had noticed two full drawers of delinquent accounts. They were stacked in as tight as could be. One day I asked the comptroller about them.

"What in the devil are you planning to do with those?"

"Oh, 90 percent of them'll go on to the collector. It'll be his headache for a change."

"Can I have a go at them first?"

"Well, Don," he hesitated, then said thoughtfully, "why not? Wait until I have a chance to discuss it with the boss."

"He says go ahead and see what you can do," the report came back the following day.

I took on the challenge. Everybody, including myself, was amazed at the results in a few weeks. Gradually that pile of delin-

amazed at the results in a few weeks. Gradually that pile of delinquent accounts shrunk to a manageable size. The boss came in to congratulate me.

When I'd been at Anktons Power Plant a full year, we decided it was time to buy some property and build a house. Our children were growing. Floyd and Toni and their six children had moved out from Minnesota. Except for fair weather times, it was impossible for us to entertain a gathering of the clan or a group of friends at Pup House.

Both Mary Ann and I liked the St. Johns area. Originally a little town, St. Johns had been incorporated as part of Portland years ago. It derived its name from the benefactor and founder, James John.

Parts of St. Johns community were run down . . . buildings deserted or sadly in need of repair, jerry-built homes left over from war days. The area had retained somewhat of a bad name dating from those days, too, because of the influx of shipyard workers and sailors from foreign ports.

But Mary Ann and I could see its potential. There was a warmth, a genuine neighborhood quality. Generations settled and stayed . . . grandparents, sons and daughters, children, aunts, uncles, and cousins. The community center was a lively place with a spacious park beside it. The center offered a year-round program of activities for all ages . . . tumbling, basketball, volley ball, drama, craft classes, sewing.

In 1931, a small boy growing up on a farm in South Dakota had no way of knowing what was going on in the St. Johns area of Portland, Oregon. A bridge was being built, a gossamer structure spanning the Willamette River. Designed by a famous engineer and bridge-builder David Steinman—who dared experiment in ways no engineer had ever experimented before—it was later declared one of the seven most beautiful bridges in the world.

At the time it was dedicated, the St. Johns bridge was the largest steel strand suspension bridge in the world. Its tall viaduct piers and 408-foot high towers had a Gothic effect that turned it into a poem of steel and concrete.

And so St. Johns had its community center, its bridge, its fire hall and police station and library, its Lombard Avenue lined with shops and restaurants and taverns, like a Main Street of a small town. Probably this is what we liked best . . . being able to be part of a city the size of Portland, yet able to preserve some of the small town flavor.

Parallel to Lombard Avenue but several blocks away, we found a piece of property for sale on a wide dirt road. We would have neighbors in the tall white house next door. It had been converted into three apartments. The lady who owned those apartments was selling us the land we wanted to buy.

"Are we really going to build our own house?" asked Nomie, wide-eyed, as we talked over our plans.

"How are you going to pay for it?" worried Greg, always very practical. "Doesn't land cost a lot of money?"

"There are loans," I told him. "Mary Ann, this is one house we're going to plan down to the last inch. We can have everything exactly as we want, and no one can tell us otherwise."

"Let's not take out a single tree," decided Mary Ann. "Look, there's a fig tree, and a pear, and an apple tree, too. Say, Don, we can leave room in the yard to plow up a bit of garden for Dad Kirkendall so he can raise a few tomatoes and corn and feel like a farmer again!"

The authorities were adamant. No loan on unimproved property. But with a little talking back and forth, we worked the deal through and gave the owner her down payment.

To our amazement, she said, "Mr. Kirkendall, why don't you buy the apartments next door, along with this lot? I want to get rid of them. I can let you have them for a very small down payment."

"Mrs. Deerfield, it was hard enough to scrape money together to cover the down payment on our land. I can't consider it."

She kept on wheedling. Exasperated, I said at last, "If I'm lucky I could manage about one hundred dollars for a down payment." I wanted to shut her up.

To my astonishment, she called up the next day. "I'll take the hundred down."

It was only a verbal contract. Because of the loan we'd taken, I could not make a legal contract. Mrs. Deerfield understood that. She considered the apartments ours.

"We've made a new investment," I chuckled to Mary Ann. "We can rent the two apartments on the top floor and, while our new home is being built, our family can live in the one below. After that we'll persuade Mom and Dad Kirkendall to move in there. I don't have to charge them a nickel, either . . . I'm so happy to find a way to repay them for some of the care they've given to me through the years."

In spite of the arguments we had with the contractor, it was a thrill to watch our house go up.

"We want the house turned around backward."

"With the back toward the street? That's a crazy idea!" The contractor looked dismayed. He eyed me curiously.

"It has nothing to do with my wheelchair. We merely like privacy."

"Maybe it's against the law. I'll have to check."

"Forget the law. It's my house and I want it backwards."

He saw he wasn't winning. He stalked off without a word, scratching his head.

Because of my wheelchair, the patio was to be graded to each door level. That patio ended up being a big headache for the contractor. He had bid too low for it so he gave it to us as a gift. At first he tried to argue me out of some of my ideas. But when he found out how stubborn I was, he called up the cement man he had subcontracted to and told him tersely, "Do whatever they want and bill me for it."

We didn't think our ideas about house-building were crazy. One thing we insisted on . . . no step on the front door. ("Not even a very shallow one?" asked the contractor). I wanted to be able to get through any door in my house without assistance. So the order remained, no step on the front door.

When our house was complete, we would have a roomy, elshaped living room opening onto the patio. Partly partitioned off from the living room would be a small but adequate kitchenette. In back of this there would be a utility room and here I insisted on another door.

"Why?" This time it was Mary Ann who asked the question.

"I have a hunch I may make my living from that room one of these days." I couldn't explain what I meant because I didn't know myself. It was just a hunch.

So a door went in on the utility room, and, because Mary Ann wanted it, another door went in on the opposite side of the house. People coming down the road would look for a door there, where the front of a normal house would usually be, she claimed, and I guess she was right.

Our home would have wide halls and no carpeting to obstruct or slow down the movement of my wheelchair. All of the doors would be cut extra wide, too, to accommodate the chair. The toilet in the bathroom would be a few inches higher than most so I could slide easily onto it. We decided to have it placed adjacent to the tub. This way it would be possible for me to ease myself out of the bath when nobody else was around. The three bedrooms opened off the hallway.

"When will our new house be done . . . oh when will it be done?" Kip danced around the patio with the same grace her mother had always had. She was a slender, bright-eyed, gifted child.

Nomie and Greg raced over the yard, exploring every corner, throwing green apples at each other until I put a stop to the game.

Mary Ann and I shared the same sense of elation. We took baths together in the downstairs apartment next door and while we scrubbed each other, we sang lustily.

Already we had new tenants in the upper rooms. "This apartment house will pay for itself," I commented to Mary Ann one night.

She nodded. "Now let me scrub your back." She slapped

on a soapy cloth and began another song. I joined her at the top of my lungs.

Halfway through it she stopped and burst out laughing. "Listen! The tenant upstairs is accompanying us on her accordian!"

We were in our house a short time when Mary Ann announced, "I want to go back to meter-maiding."

"Why, when I have such a good income now? You don't need to."

"I want to do it though," she said. "It will help pay bills. Besides . . ." she glanced around at the house ". . . I love our home but I don't picture myself devoting hours and hours a day to housework. I'm not the type."

Back she went. This time it did not seem to put her under the same physical strain so I didn't object too loudly. She knew I wanted to be the one to support our family. But I, in turn, sensed how she needed to take wing, to be apart from us somehow for a while.

Four months later, I persuaded her to give up meter-maiding forever. The day she quit, she found a surprise waiting for her at home. A new picture. One of a colorful, triumphant-looking bull with a background of mountains and a gaudy yellow sun.

"He's such a happy bull!" she said, laughing at the picture. "It's vibrant, Don . . . the bull is recognizable but you've cut him into abstract lines and planes . . . it was worth quitting my job just to receive the painting!"

My boss at Anktons had told me I could expect a bonus soon. He also hinted I was due for a raise. Things were going well, so it was a crushing blow when the owner of the power plant died and it was discovered the inheritance tax would be exorbitant. The company closed down. I found myself sitting in the living room of our new home without a job.

After I worked through the worst of my feelings, I said to Mary Ann, "I've got a good background in credit management.

I saved Anktons $72,000 on those delinquent accounts last year. I know the figure is correct because I kept track of the amount personally.''

"They thought so highly of you. Don, I'm sure you won't have any difficulty finding another job.''

I think I realized more than she did how much wheelchairs get in the way when you go job-hunting. Many people were unable to see beyond my chair. In the past I had held part-time or low-paying jobs. This was not my choice. I had flown a plane, been leader of a band, run my own radio show, studied for a year at the university, taken a course in executive bookkeeping, had eighteen months of art school, including a course in commercial art. I was raising a family of three healthy children, was in the process of buying a home and some apartments. I could drive a car and mow my own lawn with a ride-in mower.

I had, in fact, saved my last employer thousands of dollars by taking over his back accounts. But during the next three weeks, every time I made a job application I got turned down.

Twenty-nine applications. Twenty-nine rejections. Most of the applications were in the field of credit management. I had proved my skill in this area and had the course at the business college to offer as a credential.

At last a man in the employment agency told me the blunt truth, "It is the wheelchair, Donald. Nobody seems to want to take the risk of hiring a man in a wheelchair, no matter how well he can do the job.''

It was difficult, impossible almost, for me to see myself through other people's eyes. My wheelchair was as much a part of me as breath or blood. I never had considered myself a crippled little man in a chair and neither did those who knew me. Hadn't Mary Ann told me I was the most masculine man she'd ever known? She should know, having been married once to a handsome hulk of a guy six feet four inches tall who had been the hunting and fishing type.

The wheelchair was the public's hang up, not mine. Invariably, in public places, I was treated as if I was subhuman. Elevator girls would order my wife, ''Move it to the rear of the car, please.'' In restaurants, waitresses without fail set the menu in front of my wife, assuming I could not order for myself. When the bill was made out, they deposited it at her elbow, not mine. Movie houses had refused to let us in because it would be a fire hazard to have a wheelchair cluttering up the aisle. Transcontinental airplanes posed another problem. Unless I was willing to rig myself up in a complicated harness and plastic bag, there was no bathroom accommodation for a man in a wheelchair.

As a licensed driver I was unable to get regular car insurance . . . I was considered too high a risk. Instead I was part of the ''car pool.'' State law required each insurance company to take its turn giving insurance to ''a risk person.''

Health insurance too was out of the question.

''I think,'' commented Mary Ann on one occasion, ''I know what it must feel like to be black. I'm married to a minority.''

Some individuals accepted the wheelchair as an item of little significance . . . the Sealys and the Shorty Longs and the Duchesses I had encountered throughout life. People like the buxom dame at a club in Seaside who saw me staring in dismay at the long staircase leading down to the men's room while the door to the ladies lounge was conveniently located at the top of the stairs.

''You gotta go, buddy?'' she inquired. ''Wait a minute and I'll clear the place out for you.'' She flung open the door of the lounge and ordered in a commanding tone: ''OK girls, everybody out!'' To me she said, ''Go on in and take your time. I'll stand guard.''

Aside from the people who openly treated me like a mindless vegetable, I had met many who made hurting comments out of sheer thoughtlessness.

The owner of a swanky Portland department store was one of these. I went in with Mary Ann and Kip and Nomie to buy them each a coat. The owner himself happened to be on hand

and, when he saw my chair, said impatiently, "Park it over in the corner, please. It's in the way here."

"Sir, I'd like to have you know one thing," I retorted, as coolly as I could. "I am not an *it*. I am a person."

The man's face reddened. He recovered himself and, in a gracious manner, apologized. Not only that, he took time to sit down by me and chat while his salesgirls brought their finest garments to show my wife and the girls. Presently he slipped into the back room and returned bearing two glasses of his best Scotch. We sipped and talked like old friends until the three coats had been purchased.

People like this store owner and the buxom lady in the club at Seaside saved me from bitterness.

After several weeks of job-hunting, I came home and said to Mary Ann, "There's one way out. I'll start a business of my own. I've got the background to do that."

Her eyes twinkled. "Don't forget, you rated 96 percent in the persuasive arts on that test you took in college!"

"And," I reminded her, "it seems to me it was one half of 1 percent on the business part. But I've changed. Besides, credit management is largely a persuasive art."

I felt better having made a decision.

To build one's own business from the ground up . . . that is tough work. But I determined I would succeed.

"I told you I'd be making a living from our utility room one day. It was a hunch. . . ."

Mary Ann and Jack's wife, Laurie, had agreed to be my part-time clerks. I would need Mary Ann to do much of the legwork for me, visiting doctors and clinics and dentists to see about delinquent accounts.

My clientele built up at a slow pace. First I approached our family doctor, told him my background, and asked if he'd be interested in having me handle his delinquent accounts. Without hesitation, he agreed. Next a drugstore owner became interest- ed, and then another doctor, and the manager of a grocery store.

As yet I had no operator's license. I could not legitimately call myself a Collector so I didn't need to have a trust account set up or to be bonded. Most important, I was careful not to handle any of the money that came in. Every bit of the cash and all the checks bypassed my office and went directly to the clients who had hired me.

I was eager to get my operator's license as soon as possible. I studied and failed the test.

Discouraged, I complained, "Those questions are so ambiguous . . . I think I'll ask my attorney friend, Dave Murdock, to help me on some of the harder points of law."

I made out a long list of questions. Dave stopped by our house on his way home from work and answered them patiently, one by one. Another lawyer coached me on the universal commercial code, a new design to make all states as equal as possible in matters of civil law.

While I was studying, Dad entered the hospital for surgery. He was an old old man but this was a minor malady. He came over to visit me before he left. He sounded as brusque as ever when he said, "One of these days I'll go, son. But I don't want you boys to feel bad about it. Son of a bitch, I've lived a pretty good life. . . ."

The day before I was to take the test my father died.

"Whaddya know!" I exclaimed softly when I heard the news. "He and I were just talking about that a while ago."

My father had taught me not to be afraid of change, not to give in, above all, to be myself instead of striving to be a carbon copy of someone I admired. With his passing, one of the greatest influences of my life was gone.

("Let me hoist you up on the haymow, son . . . there now, as I was saying, the year I worked in Canada. . . . Son of a bitch, here comes that preacher man . . . just tell him I've gone to Woonsocket. . . . You'll make it, Don, I know you will. . . .")

"You know what I found when I was going through Kirk's

211

belongings?'' Mom's lip trembled. ''The papers on the Drake Estate.''

I looked at them with curiosity . . . faded, yellow, worthless papers. They symbolized Dad's trust in humanity. When I returned the papers to Mom I saw her fold them and tuck them carefully back into the drawer of her desk.

I felt a sense of loss, as if something were finished . . . a life that would not be again. But I cannot say I grieved. I felt happy to recall how proud my father had been of my successes in marriage and family and business. I, too, had achieved a fulfillment in being able to support him in his last years. And he died knowing his wife, my mother, would live comfortably and well cared for until the end of her days.

The small boy they once feared might be dependent upon others had grown to the full stature of manhood.

Both Father John and his brother, Father Con Hooyber, stopped what they were doing and attended the funeral. A Mormon sang and an Episcopalian conducted the service.

I took the test for my operator's license and, once again, I failed. It made me even more determined to make the grade. Three months must pass before I would be permitted to take it again so I had time to study.

The third time I received a letter of congratulations and a license. I could call myself a full-fledged Collection Agency at last! The license did not mean that business would pick up in a hurry. Many months we were so poor that I wondered if I could go on.

Dad came to mind . . . his grit . . . his way of never giving up.

By now I had formed some deep friendships within the St. Johns community. One of these, a local photographer, Owen Mossbarger, could pull me out of a funky mood better than anyone else.

''I went through the same thing,'' he'd say in his mild but winning way. ''When I first went into business for myself it seemed as if I'd never make it. But you know what, Don? If you hang on it'll get better. You hardly know it's happening but it will . . . Don't give up!''

Owen was right. My monthly wages swelled gradually until I was making a livable income. Even before this happened, I went out and bought myself a used Cadillac.

"Why?" Mary Ann couldn't help asking. To her it looked too flashy, somebody in our financial state doing such a thing. "We can't afford it, Don. How are you going to pay for it?"

"I'll find a way, don't you worry."

The Cadillac spurred me to work like a demon. Within ninety days I covered its entire cost—$500—and had money left over for our food.

I joined the St. Johns Boosters and, in time, I received an invitation to join North Portland Rotary. At first my motive for participating in both clubs was purely selfish . . . the contact with other merchants would enable me to become better known and my business would expand. But I soon discovered I was becoming interested in civic affairs.

Mary Ann had been taking the dance course offered by the city bureau of parks and recreation. Now she was ready to offer something of her own creative talent. She would be teaching dance drama at the St. Johns Community Center. Nomie and Kip participated. Greg was far more interested in meetings of the Civil Air Patrol. As soon as he graduated from high school he joined the Marines.

It startled me to watch him go. Time had played a trick on me. Was this Shorty Long or Jack or Floyd taking off so jauntily in uniform? Where was the tow-headed kid who had shot arrows from the windows of the play shack out in back of Pup House? Where was the small boy gloating over his closet bedroom? Greg . . . come back to me . . . But he was gone.

Years ago, my brother Jack had vowed neither he nor any member of his family would ride in a car when I was at the wheel.

But when Laurie called me in the middle of the night in tears, it was I who got dressed as quickly as I could and rushed him to the hospital. He had been stricken with a heart attack.

"These things run in our family," Jack warned me when he was convalescing. "You better take a hint and slow down, Don. You're going along at quite a clip you know."

"Can't help it. Life is just too full." I had been elected to the board of North Portland Rotary. I was secretary of the St. Johns Booster Club. My business was flourishing. I had invested in six more apartments and a new yellow convertible—the first brand-spanking new car I'd ever owned in my life.

And then Jack's words came true. At the age of forty-three I, too, was laid low by a major heart attack. Mary Ann kept her terror to herself. She took care of business matters and the family. She continued to teach her dance course. Never once did she look flustered when she came to the hospital to visit. As I began to recover, she and I discussed the hospital bill. It would be enormous because my wheelchair prevented me from being eligible for any hospitalization plan.

"The doctor tells me you could be moved to the county hospital," Mary Ann suggested one day. "You'd receive good care there and the cost would be minimal."

Already, in two short weeks, we owed over two thousand dollars worth of medical expenses!

Once I was settled in the county hospital, Mary Ann brought me my electric wheelchair. I could be out of bed for a short time every day. One afternoon she found me at the opposite end of the corridor in another patient's room. She burst out laughing.

"For goodness' sakes, Don, the nurses are complaining that they can't keep up with you! Heart attacks are serious business. If you can't slow down, I'd better take that chair back home with me." In the midst of her distress she was able to joke like that, but I sensed her laughter was tinged with tears. She thought of me as a vibrant personality. It hurt her to see me down.

Before I went home the doctor gave me a prescription nobody could fill but myself.

"You need to sweep the cobwebs from your mind, Don. Your business is too exacting. Cut down the work and get outside and do something new and different. Get some exercise."

He studied my electric wheelchair. "I do mean exercise. If it was anybody else, I'd say do a lot of walking. But I've noticed how much effort it takes to get in and out of that chair. And I imagine you spend a good deal more energy while you're actually riding in it. So get out and take long rides in it instead of sitting at home in the office."

"As a matter of fact, you guessed correctly," I told him. "Most people don't realize how much energy my chair uses up. I'd like to see anyone else try it out on rough terrain. It has absolutely no spring action, so even while I'm sitting down, my body is moving every bit of the time."

I thought about what I would do to fill his prescription. Something new and different. Why not run for state representative?

"You're wild!" exclaimed Mary Ann gleefully. "But why not? Campaigning will get us outside, moving around. We'll meet loads of new people and have a good time doing it."

Neither of us felt North Portland was adequately represented by the incumbent. I prepared my platform. During the late summer and early fall, whenever I could tear myself away from my office, Mary Ann and I campaigned for Kirkendall. We talked to important people. We went into the poverty pockets. I was continually bombarded with questions, confronted by men and women and young people eager to find ways to bring about change. Portland had experienced the rumblings of a racial riot this very summer. It had been quelled within a few days, but not until several buildings had been burned and tension had mounted to the breaking point. What was I going to do about that, people wanted to know. What was I going to do about that?

When election day rolled around in November I did not win a place as state representative. But I had achieved my private purpose of clearing the cobwebs out of my head and doing something new.

Until now I had never considered myself a political animal.

Campaigning had shown me the importance of developing personal political power if I hoped to bring about change in my community. I could not remain a nobody if I wanted to do that.

And I wasn't a nobody anymore.

Mary Ann and I had ordered a trailer custom-built to accommodate my wheelchair. Our family still loved to camp. The new trailer gave us an opportunity to take long trips with ease. We went to California and, one spring, as far away as Mexico.

I accepted the job of Parade Chairman for the St. Johns Day Parade. This turned out to be an enormous task of organization but my heart attack was two years in the past. I had regained strength and tackled the task with vigor.

Three weeks after the parade I suffered a second heart attack. This time I told Mary Ann, "When I recover, I'm going to hire some extra help at the office. Maybe my life will be shorter than some, but I've got a lot of living left to do and I'm going to do it!"

I was forty-five years old.

---

## fourteen

I saw Portland as it was and I saw it as it could be. Some parts of the city were expanding, other parts were dying off. The city had a staff of hard-working officials but, like other growing cities, there was a communications gap which needed to be closed. The mayor had formed a task force of citizens for this express purpose.

Like most other places, Portland was designed for people sound of limb. How about the others . . . veteran amputees returning from Vietnam, children born with congenital defects, men and women suffering from strokes or severe heart conditions or diseases like multiple sclerosis? How about those crippled by auto accidents?

How could they go up and down church and library steps? How could they go to school? (''We're sorry, Mr. and Mrs. Kirkendall, we've come to tell you your son will not be able to attend high school . . .'' ''Where is the men's room? Downstairs in the lounge, of course . . .''

217

I was not a veteran, attempting suddenly to get used to moving about on wheels. I had lived that way for over forty years. All my life I had noticed simple changes that could be made . . .

At a meeting of the Boosters I suggested curb cuts in the St. Johns area.

Curb cuts? What are they? You cut out the curb at the street corner, making it similar to any driveway . . . and so a wheelchair can cross the street without a problem.

Today St. Johns has curb cuts.

In the early sixties, Portland gained a famous shopping center, the Lloyd Center. It is the easiest place in town for wheelchair users to shop—dozens and dozens of department stores, restaurants, banks, beauty parlors, photo shops, book stores, and health food stores opening off the mall. Nothing but pedestrian traffic, and large parking lots at the back of the Center and in underground tiers.

Much more is being done today, across the country, to eliminate architectural barriers. Because of the influx of returned veterans, many with permanent physical disabilities, universities are now amply supplied with ramps. In some cities special buses are designated for wheelchairs. These vehicles are equipped with a hydraulic lift to get the chairs into the bus. Those chairs without brakes have a safety strap snapped around their wheels to render them immobile in transit.

Churches and other public buildings have put in ramps. The Oregon Museum of Science and Industry has one built into the middle of its concrete steps.

This is a beginning.

After running a successful business for ten years, I decided to retire. Kip was in high school, Nomie and Greg were married, and Mary Ann had entered her second year as one of the Directors of the St. Johns Community Center. Some of the investments I had made were bringing in a steady income. And there was so much I wanted to do besides running a Collection Agency.

I sold my accounts, with the agreement that, for the next five years, I would be a silent partner in the business, receiving 25 percent of the gross income from those particular accounts.

Later I might decide I wanted to work part time, or even full time again, at a different job. Right now I had plenty of income from these varied sources. And I had other things to keep me busy.

I was the newly elected president of the St. Johns Boosters, and also the president of the North Portland Citizens Committee. And, too, I was playing one of the the central character parts in a play the drama group at the Community Center had written and produced under my wife's direction. But there was something else on my mind.

I called up my old friend, the mayor. "I've been reading about the task force you've appointed to study the problems of the city . . . Terry, that's something I'd like to do."

"Fine," he told me. "I hereby appoint you a member of the force."

One of the major concerns of Portland residents, especially those working on committees in the northern area, was the Columbia River slough. Stretching for seven miles near the point where the Columbia and the Willamette meet, the slough had become a stinking mess of sewage. There was a continual tangle between the Port of Portland which wanted to clean it up and reserve it for small boating and recreational purposes, and industries that hoped to dredge it and use it in a commercial way.

Along with sewage emptying into the murky water, the oozing banks were an eyesore, littered with old rubber tires, broken bottles, rusty bedsprings, shingles, and cans.

Because I had held various local civic offices, people kept asking me questions about the slough. What was my opinion? What did I think should be done?

I wanted to find out more about it. How could I discuss the problem intelligently unless I did some firsthand investigation?

I had an idea.

During the summer I had worked on a new project, taking

219

documentary film of the St. Johns community, paying special attention to the section around and under the bridge. We were working toward the formation of a new park, Cathedral Park, so called because of the stunning patterns cast by the lights and shadows of the bridge's gothic spires.

I consulted authorities at the Port of Portland.

"We need to interest the public to a point where they'll insist on action. How? Articles in the newspaper? Yes, but more than that . . . pictures. I could make a movie documentary. Shown around the city it might have a galvanic effect."

"That's a great idea. We can have someone take you out there in a pickup with four wheel drive. That way you can see things at close range."

The film turned out fine. As the authorities watched it, a voice spoke up: "We should get some more pictures from a helicopter."

"If you'll provide the 'copter, I'll go up."

"I'll hire one for you, Don." It was the executive director of the Port of Portland who was speaking now.

In a day he called me on the telephone. "I've lined up a helicopter. Would one thirty Tuesday afternoon be all right? One of our men, Joel Ruby, will go with you."

A city commissioner telephoned about another matter. "I'm told you're the man who went down to Salem and appeared before the subcommittee at the state legislature to help push through the bill on doing away with architectural barriers. We're designating special funds to try this out in a test area in downtown Portland. Would you be willing to advise us? In some places ramps may work better than the curb cuts you have out there in St. Johns. But of course they might interfere with water drainage into the street during stormy weather. We'll be working closely with an engineer. Later we expect to undertake a massive program . . . no reason the entire city can't be made accessible to all of its citizens. . . ."

"Sure . . . I'll do what I can."

"We'll send a girl out to interview you. We've hired students to make an extensive survey."

The girl was young, college age, intent on her project. She asked many questions.

"Occupation?"

"Retired. At least for now."

She flashed me a reassuring smile. Did I detect a note of sympathy? (Can't you see it isn't because of my wheelchair, this early retirement . . . I have many things to do and so little time . . . Who knows what I may be doing next year . . . something new and different . . . something I've never done before.)

More questions. Pages of them.

"We're almost done, Mr. Kirkendall. Thank you for cooperating. Just one more question. What was the last form of public transportation you used?"

I knew she must be thinking of the buses in a few of our larger cities . . . the ones rigged up with hydraulic lifts and reserved for wheelchairs. Portland has none of these. The community college has minibuses though, to carry wheelchair users back and forth to classes.

I thought about the movie I had made of the slough . . . three of us up in the air. . . . ("Hang on to my belt and back brace, Joel . . . real tight now while I lean out to take some pictures. Hold on tight . . . here we go!")

Don't categorize me, I wanted to say to the girl. Please don't pigeonhole me as a handicapped person.

"Mr. Kirkendall," she repeated, "what was the last form of public transportation you used?"

"A helicopter," I told her, enjoying the look of astonishment on her face. "One rented for me by the Port of Portland."

She packed up her notebook and ballpoint pen and fled.

221

I am Don Kirkendall. A person. Limited in some ways by a wheelchair. Perhaps.

"She wanted to know why I retired early," I said to Mary Ann that night.

"And what did you tell her?" she asked sleepily.

"Oh . . . I needed time to do the things I want to do."

"Like what?"

"Like going on a special honeymoon with you . . . does British Columbia interest you? Or San Francisco? Or Reno? And other things. . . . ."

"What things?"

"Some day I'd like to race a stock car."